THE MEDITERRANEAN ON THE PLATE

A 360° Cookbook for a Deep Immersion Inside The Gastronomic Mediterranean Tradition for Long Term Health Benefits

Mediterranean Flavor

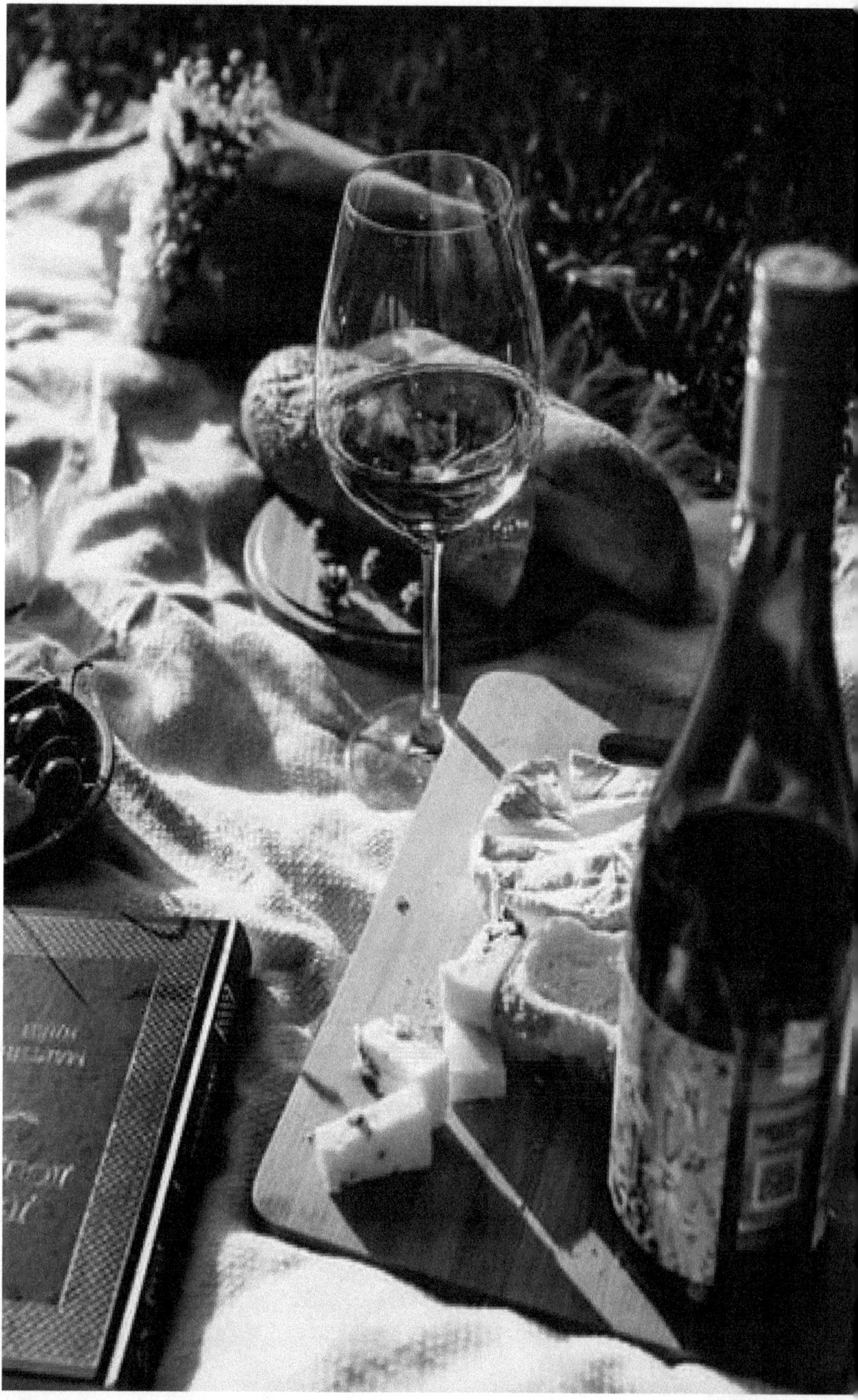

the publisher or the original author of this work can be in any fashion deemed liable for any hardship or damages that may befall them after undertaking the information described herein.

Additionally, the information in the following pages is intended only for informational purposes and should thus be thought of as universal. As befitting its nature, it is presented without assurance regarding its prolonged validity or interim quality. Trademarks that are mentioned are done without written consent and can in no way be considered an endorsement from the trademark holder.

Table of Contents

INTRODUCTION

The Mediterranean Diet is the traditional diet of the countries surrounding the Mediterranean Sea, such as Greece, Spain, and Italy. It focuses on the regional foods from those countries, which have many benefits, including improving heart health, chronic disease, and obesity.

The Mediterranean Diet reflects the personality of these regions and includes a wonderful variety of ingredients and recipes, featuring grains, fats from fish, olive oil, nuts, fruits, and lean meats. It is easy to follow and will provide lots of healthy and delicious meals that your family will love.

This diet is generally characterized by a high intake of plant-based food such as fresh fruits, vegetables, nuts and cereals, and olive oil, with a moderate amount of fish and poultry, and a small amount of dairy products, red meats, and sweets. Wine is allowed with every meal but at a moderate level. The Mediterranean Diet focuses strongly on social and cultural activities like communal mealtimes, resting after eating, and physical activities.

The Mediterranean Diet is not simply a weight loss or fad diet; however, raising your dietary fiber and cutting down on red meat, animal fats, and processed foods will lead to weight loss and a decreased risk of many diseases.

The Mediterranean Diet Pyramid

The Mediterranean Diet Pyramid is a visual tool that summarizes the diet. It suggests pattern of eating and gives guidelines for meal frequency and food management. This pyramid allows you to develop healthy eating habits and maintain calorie counts as well.

The pyramid tiers consist of the following groups:

- **Plant-based foods**

This includes olive oil, fruits, vegetables, whole grains, legumes, beans, nuts and seeds, and spices and herbs. These foods should be part of every meal. Olive oil is the main fat used in cooking. It can occasionally be replaced with butter or cooking oil, but in smaller quantities.

Fresh herbs and spices can be used in generous amounts in dishes for enhancing taste and as an alternative to salt. Dried herbs can also be used. Fresh ginger and garlic are always allowed for flavor.

- **Seafood**

Seafood is an important staple and one of the main sources of protein in the Mediterranean Diet. Make sure you have seafood at least twice a week. There are many varieties of fish that will work, as well as mussels, shrimps, and crab. Tuna is a great source of protein and works well in sandwiches and salads.

- **Dairy and Poultry**

Yogurt, milk, cheese, and poultry can be consumed at a moderate level. If you use eggs in cooking and baking, include them in your weekly limit. Choose healthy cheese options like ricotta, feta, and parmesan. You can have them as toppings and garnishing your meals and dishes.

- **Sweets and Red Meat**

Sweets and meats are used less in this diet. If you eat them, cut down on the quantity and choose lean meat. Red meat, sugar, and fat are not good for heart health and blood sugar.

- **Water**

The Mediterranean Diet encourages increased daily water intake, 9 8-ounce glasses for women and 13 for men. For pregnant and breastfeeding women, the amount should be higher.

- **Wine**

The Mediterranean Diet allows for moderate wine consumption with meals. Alcohol reduces the risk of heart disease. One glass of wine for women and two for men is the recommended daily limit.

Foods That Are Not Allowed in the Mediterranean Diet

This diet satisfies your food cravings by providing better alternatives. It helps you to shift your mindset from looking for snacks to having fresh fruits and vegetables that will satisfy your between-meal hunger.

The following items should be restricted or replaced by healthy options:

- **Added sugar**

Sugar is one of the most difficult items to avoid in your diet. Try to stick to healthy sugar from fresh fruits and vegetables. Avoid processed foods; the added sugars in pasta sauce, peanut butter, fruit juices, bread, and bakery products are considered empty calories.

Added sugars are commonly used in processed food like:

- High fructose corn syrup
- Glucose
- Corn syrup

- Sucrose
- Maltose
- Corn sweetener

You can add fresh fruits like strawberries and raspberries to your water for flavor and refreshment as well as eating them. Switch to an organic sweetener like honey or maple syrup instead of using refined sugars.

- **Refined grains**

Refined grains are prohibited in the Mediterranean Diet because they lead to heart disease and type 2 diabetes. Grains are often grouped with carbohydrates, but they do not fall into the "bad carbs" category until they are refined. Refined grains go through a milling process during which the major nutrients are removed. They are left with less fiber, iron, and vitamins and more empty calories.

The most common refined grains consist of:

- White flour
- White bread
- White rice
- White flour pizza crust

- **Breakfast cereals**

Whole grains are a better alternative. When possible, choose sourdough bread. Enjoy sandwiches in a whole-grain wrap or pita bread. You can also try plant-based alternatives like cauliflower crust, cauliflower rice, or spiralized vegetables in place of pasta. Swap in whole grains like quinoa and brown rice.

- **Refined Oils**

Refined oils are extremely damaging to your health. The key nutrients have been stripped from out and additional chemicals added in, making their way to your food.

Most oils are extracted from the seeds of plants. This includes soybean oil, corn oil, sunflower oil, peanut oil, and olive oil. Vegetable oils are a combination of multiple plants. The process of extracting the oil involves a variety of chemicals that can increase inflammation in the body. The fat that remains in the oil has been linked to several health conditions such as cancer, heart disease, and diabetes. Oils are also used to create margarine in a hydrogenation process, using chemicals that allow the oil to remain in a solid-state. When the oil is hydrogenated, the fatty acids that were in the oil are further destroyed and transformed into trans fatty acids. Several scientific studies have been conducted to show the connection of trans fatty acids to some debilitating health conditions.

Trans fatty acids are considered to be some of the unhealthiest fats you can consume, especially when it comes to your heart. These industrially manufactured fats cause LDL cholesterol to increase. High amounts of LDL or bad cholesterol can clog and destroy your arteries and increase blood pressure. This significantly increases your risk of heart attack and stroke.

Some of the most common trans fats or hydrogenated oils that you might not be aware of include:

- Microwaveable popcorn
- Butter
- Margarine
- Vegetable oil
- Fried foods
- Pre-packaged muffins, cakes, doughnuts, and pastries
- Coffee creamers
- Prepared pizza dough or pizza crust
- Cake frosting
- Potato chips
- Crackers

The Mediterranean Diet focuses on replacing these refined oils and processed foods with more wholesome and natural ingredients. Refined oils can be easy to eliminate from your diet. If you are used to sautéing your foods with refined oil, switch to unrefined olive oil. Instead of frying foods in oil, bake or grill them.

- **Processed Meat**

Processed meats have been processed extensively to preserve flavors and provide a longer shelf life. The most common forms are bacon, hot dogs, deli meats, sausage, and canned meats. Consuming processed meat daily can cause or increase the risk of colorectal cancer, stomach cancer, pancreatic cancer, and prostate cancer.

Sodium is what makes processed meats so harmful. Sodium is well known to increase blood pressure, which increases the risk of different heart diseases. Processed meat contains at least 50 percent more preservatives than unprocessed meats. These preservatives affect sugar tolerances and can cause insulin resistance, which can lead to diabetes.

- Switch out processed meats and red meats for fish or poultry.
- Use vegetables or beans in place of meat.

- Use a variety of spices to add more flavor to a dish where you would use meat in the same way.
- Spices like cumin, coriander, peppercorn, and marjoram add unique flavors to the dish so you won't miss the bacon, sausage, or ground meat.
- You can use different seasonings on sautéed or baked vegetables.
- Add roasted chickpeas or toasted seeds and nuts to dishes for more texture. These can be great alternatives to dishes that call for bacon crumbles.

Common Mistakes in the Mediterranean Diet:

When you start a new diet, you will make some mistakes or encounter situations in which you don't know what to do. Before you get on the Mediterranean Diet plan, here is a heads-up about common mistakes that people make. If you know about these mistakes, you can avoid them and achieve success more quickly.

- **All or Nothing**

Your attitude toward your diet matters a lot. This is why you must make sure you are mentally prepared for it. It will be different from your ordinary lifestyle, which is why you need an abundance of information. To learn the benefits of this diet, you can ask the experts or people who have experienced it.

- **Eating the Same Things**

Don't eat the same things over and over again, day after day. One of the most common mistakes people make is that they think that eating the same kind of vegetables all week long will help them lose weight. You must have variety in your diet. The Mediterranean Diet allows you to have multiple kinds of dishes throughout the week, but maintain portion control.

- **Deprivation**

Another mistake people make is thinking that deprivation is the only way to lose weight. The main point of this diet plan is to give you energy while helping you lose weight. Deprivation will only make you weaker. This diet plan won't work if you don't eat at all, so be sure to keep this in mind.

- **Giving up**

Don't give up in the middle of the Mediterranean Diet. If you see yourself losing weight and you think, *now I can cheat a little* ... resist. Since you've put so much effort into it already, don't give up now. If you have chocolate cravings, find a healthy alternative. It's easier to develop self-control if you can see the results, so keep your goals in mind and stay strong. Our bodies need time to adjust and stabilize in terms of the food we eat, so switching back and forth is never a good option.

- **Not setting goals**

One of the main mistakes people make is not setting goals when they start the diet. You must have a goal in terms of how much weight you want to lose and work toward it. When you don't have a plan, you will become distracted and be unable to reach your destination, no matter how hard you try.

- **Following the wrong plan**

Another common mistake is that you don't have enough knowledge about the plan you are following to lose weight. Maybe you are following the wrong plan, one that doesn't seem to work for you. If you're confused, don't decide by yourself to follow the Mediterranean Diet; consult an expert who can advise you on what to eat and do to adopt a healthy lifestyle. Many people try to keep their old habits while mixing in elements of the Mediterranean Diet, but if you don't follow the diet, you won't achieve the optimal results. Decide if you're willing to do it, and then do it right.

Your Mediterranean Shopping Guide

Apart from knowing how to start your diet, it is necessary to know a little about how to set-up your food charts.

What to have:

- Fresh vegetables: tomatoes, kale, spinach, cauliflower, Brussels sprouts, cucumbers, etc.
- Fresh fruits: An orange, apples, pears, grapes, dates, strawberries, figs, peaches, etc.
- Seeds and nuts: almonds, walnuts, cashews, sunflower seeds, etc.
- Legumes: beans, lentils, chickpeas, etc.
- Roots: yams, turnips, sweet potatoes, etc.
- Whole grains: whole oats, rye, brown rice, corn, barley, buckwheat, whole wheat, whole grain pasta, and bread
- Fish and seafood: sardines, salmon, tuna, shrimp, mackerel, oyster, crab, clams, mussels, etc.
- Poultry: turkey, chicken, duck, etc.
- Eggs—chicken, duck, quail
- Dairy products such as cheese, Greek yogurt, etc.

- Herbs and spices: mint, basil, garlic, rosemary, cinnamon, sage, pepper, etc.
- Healthy fats and oil: extra virgin olive oil, avocado oil, olives, etc.

What to avoid:

- Foods with added sugar like soda, ice cream, candy, table sugar, etc.
- Refined grains like white bread or pasta made with refined wheat
- Margarine and similar processed foods that contain trans fats
- Refined oil such as cottonseed oil, soybean oil, etc.
- Processed meat such as hot dogs, sausages, bacon, etc.
- Highly processed food with labels such as "Low-Fat" or "Diet," or anything that is not natural

Useful Information about Healthy Foods

1. Oils

The Mediterranean Diet emphasizes healthy oils. The following are some of the oils that you might want to consider.

- **Coconut oil:** Coconut oil is semi-solid at room temperature and can be used for months without turning sour. Coconut oil also has a lot of health benefits as lauric acid, which can help to improve cholesterol levels and kill various pathogens.

- **Extra-virgin olive oil:** Olive oil is well-known worldwide as one of the healthiest oils, and it is a key ingredient in the Mediterranean Diet. Olive oil can help to improve health biomarkers such as increasing HDL cholesterol and lowering the amount of bad LDL cholesterol.

- **Avocado oil:** Avocado oil is very similar to olive oil and has similar health benefits. It can be used for many purposes as an alternative to olive oil (such as in cooking).

2. Healthy salt alternatives and spices

Aside from replacing healthy oils, the Mediterranean Diet will allow you to opt for healthy salt alternatives as well.

- **Sunflower seeds**

Sunflower seeds are excellent and give a nutty and sweet flavor.

- **Fresh squeezed lemon**

Lemon is packed with Vitamin C, which helps to neutralize damaging free radicals from the system.

- **Onion powder**

Onion powder is a dehydrated ground spice made from an onion bulb, which is mostly used as a seasoning and is a fine salt alternative.

- **Black pepper**

Black pepper is also a salt alternative that is native to India. It is made by grinding whole peppercorns.

- **Cinnamon**

Cinnamon is well-known as a savory spice and available in two varieties: Ceylon and Chinese. Both of them sport a sharp, warm, and sweet flavor.

- **Fruit-infused vinegar**

Fruit-infused vinegar or flavored vinegar can give a nice flavor to meals. These are excellent ingredients to add a bit of flavor to meals without salt.

Eating Out on the Mediterranean Diet

It might seem a bit confusing, but eating out at a restaurant while on a Mediterranean Diet is pretty easy. Just follow the simple rules below:

- Try to ensure that you choose seafood or fish as the main dish of your meal
- When ordering, try to make a special request and ask the restaurant to fry their food using extra virgin olive oil
- Ask for only whole-grain based ingredients if possible
- If possible, try to read the menu before going to the restaurant
- Try to have a simple snack before you go out; this will help prevent you from overeating.

BREAKFAST

Cheesy Mushroom egg Casserole

5 Servings

Preparation Time: 25 minutes

Ingredients

- 1 ½ oz cheddar cheese, shredded
- 1½ teaspoons canola oil
- 1 cup mushrooms, chopped
- 1 yellow onion, diced
- 5 eggs, beaten
- 1½ tablespoons coconut flakes
- 1 teaspoon chili pepper

Directions

- Add canola oil into the pan and preheat well.
- Add in mushrooms and onion and roast for 5-8 minutes or until the vegetables are light brown.
- Transfer the cooked vegetables into the casserole mold.
- Add in coconut flakes, chili pepper, and Cheddar cheese.
- Then add in eggs and stir well.
- Bake the casserole for 15 minutes at 360F

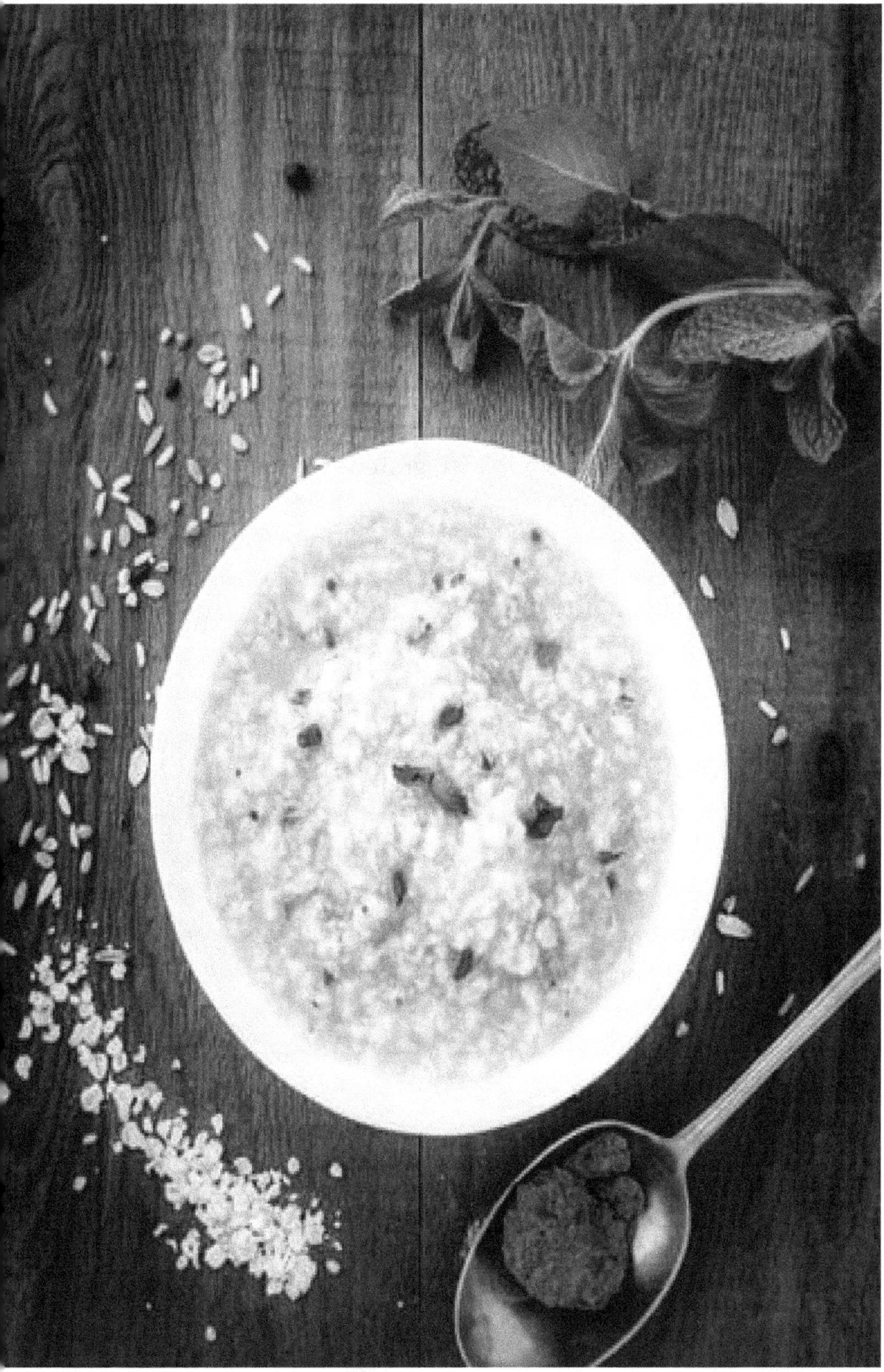

Fresh Veggies with Brown Rice Salad

6 Servings

Preparation Time: 10 minutes

Ingredients

- A pinch of salt and black pepper
- 2 tablespoons lemon juice
- ¼ teaspoon lemon zest, grated
- ¼ cup olive oil
- 9 ounces brown rice, cooked
- 7 cups baby arugula
- 15 ounces canned garbanzo beans, drained and rinsed
- 4 ounces feta cheese, crumbled
- ¾ cup basil, chopped

Directions

- In a salad bowl, combine the brown rice with the arugula, the beans, and the rest of the ingredients, toss and serve cold for breakfast.

Classical Olive and Milk Bread

8 Servings

Preparation Time: 50 minutes

Ingredients

- 1½ teaspoons baking powder
- 3 cups of wheat flour, whole grain
- 4 eggs, beaten
- 1½ teaspoons butter, melted
- 1½ cups black olives, pitted, chopped
- 1½ tablespoons olive oil
- 1 teaspoon fresh yeast
- 1 cup milk, preheated
- 1 teaspoon salt

Directions

- In the big bowl, combine together fresh yeast, sugar, and milk. Stir it until yeast is dissolved.
- Then add salt, baking powder, butter, and eggs. Stir the dough mixture and add 1 cup of wheat flour. Mix it up until smooth.
- Add olives and remaining flour. Knead the non-sticky dough.
- Transfer the dough into the non-sticky dough mold.
- Bake the bread for 50 minutes at 350 F.

- Check if the bread is cooked with the help of the toothpick. If it is dry, the bread is cooked.
- Remove the bread from the oven and let it chill for 10-15 minutes.
- Remove it from the loaf mold and slice.

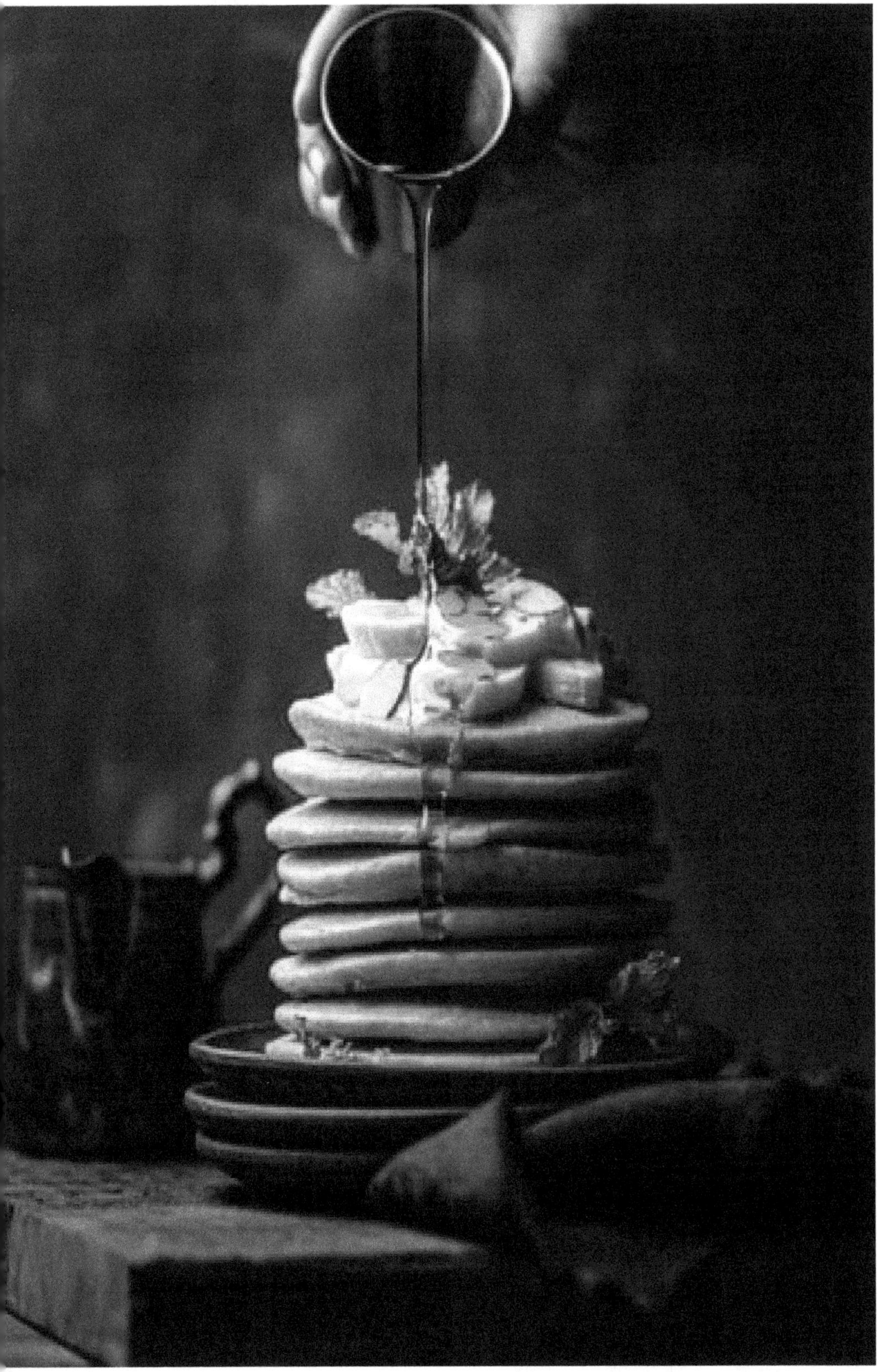

Breakfast Light Tostadas

8 Servings

Preparation Time: 6 minutes

Ingredients

- 1½ tablespoons canola oil
- 3 oz Cheddar cheese, shredded
- 1 cup white beans, canned, drained
- 8 eggs
- 1 teaspoon butter
- 1 teaspoon Sea salt
- 1 white onion, diced
- 1½ tomatoes, chopped
- 1½ cucumbers, chopped
- 1½ tablespoons fresh cilantro, chopped
- 1 jalapeno pepper, chopped
- 1½ tablespoons lime juice
- 8 corn tortillas

Directions

- Make Pico de Galo: in the salad bowl, combine together diced white onion, tomato, cucumber, fresh cilantro, and jalapeno pepper.
- Then add in lime juice and a ½ tablespoon of canola oil. Mix up the mixture well. Pico de Galo is cooked.

- Preheat the oven to 390°F.
- Line the tray with baking paper.
- Arrange the corn tortillas on the baking paper and brush with remaining canola oil from both sides.
- Bake the tortillas for 10 minutes.
- Chill the cooked crunchy tortillas well.
- Mix the butter in the pan.
- Crack the eggs in the melted butter and sprinkle them with sea salt.
- Fry the eggs until the egg whites become white (cooked). Approximately for 3-5 minutes over medium heat.
- After this, mash the beans until you get a puree texture.
- Spread the bean puree on the corn tortillas.
- Add fried eggs.
- Then top the eggs with Pico de Galo and shredded Cheddar cheese.

Chicken Souvlaki with Feta

6 Servings

Preparation Time: 12 minutes

Ingredients

- 1 cup cucumber, peeled, chopped
- 1 cup (2 ounces) feta cheese, crumbled
- 1½ tablespoons olive oil, extra-virgin, divided
- 1½ tablespoons fresh dill, chopped
- 1½ cups iceberg lettuce, shredded
- 1 teaspoon minced garlic, bottled, divided
- 6 pieces (6-inch) pitas, cut into halves
- 3 cups roasted chicken breast skinless, boneless, and sliced
- 1 cup red onion, thinly sliced
- 1 teaspoon dried oregano
- 1 cup Greek yogurt, plain
- 1 cup plum tomato, chopped

Directions

- In a small mixing bowl, combine the yogurt, cheese, 1 teaspoon of olive oil, and 1/4 teaspoon of the garlic until well mixed.
- In a large pan, heat the remaining olive oil over medium-high heat. Add the remaining 1 teaspoon garlic and the oregano cook for 20 seconds.

- Add the chicken; cook for about 2 minutes or until the chicken are heated through.
- Put 1/4 cup in chicken into each pita halves. Top with 2 tablespoons yogurt mixture, 2 tablespoons lettuce, 1 tablespoon tomato, and 1 tablespoon cucumber. Divide the onion between the pita halves.

Toasted Pine Nuts Tahini

2 Servings

Preparation Time: 10 minutes

Ingredients

- 3 teaspoons feta cheese, crumbled
- Juice of1 lemon
- 3 teaspoons pine nuts
- A pinch of black pepper
- 3 whole wheat bread slices, toasted
- 1½ teaspoons water
- 1½ tablespoons tahini paste

Directions

- In a bowl, mix the tahini with the water and the lemon juice, whisk really well, and spread over the toasted bread slices.
- Top each serving with the remaining ingredients and serve for breakfast.

Eggs with Veggies breakfast

6 Servings

Preparation Time: 15 minutes

Ingredients

- 1½ teaspoons butter
- 1 white onion, diced
- 1 teaspoon chili flakes
- 1 teaspoon sea salt
- 3 tomatoes, chopped
- 3 eggs, beaten
- 1½ bell peppers, chopped
- 1½ teaspoons of tomato paste
- 1 cup of water

Directions

- Add butter into the pan and melt it.
- Add in bell pepper and cook it for 3 minutes over medium heat. Stir it from time to time.
- Add diced onion and cook it for 2 minutes more.
- Stir in the vegetables and add tomatoes.
- Cook them for 5 minutes over medium-low heat.
- Then add water and tomato paste. Stir well.
- Add beaten eggs, chili flakes, and sea salt.
- Stir well and cook menemen for 4 minutes over medium-low heat.
- The cooked meal should be half runny.

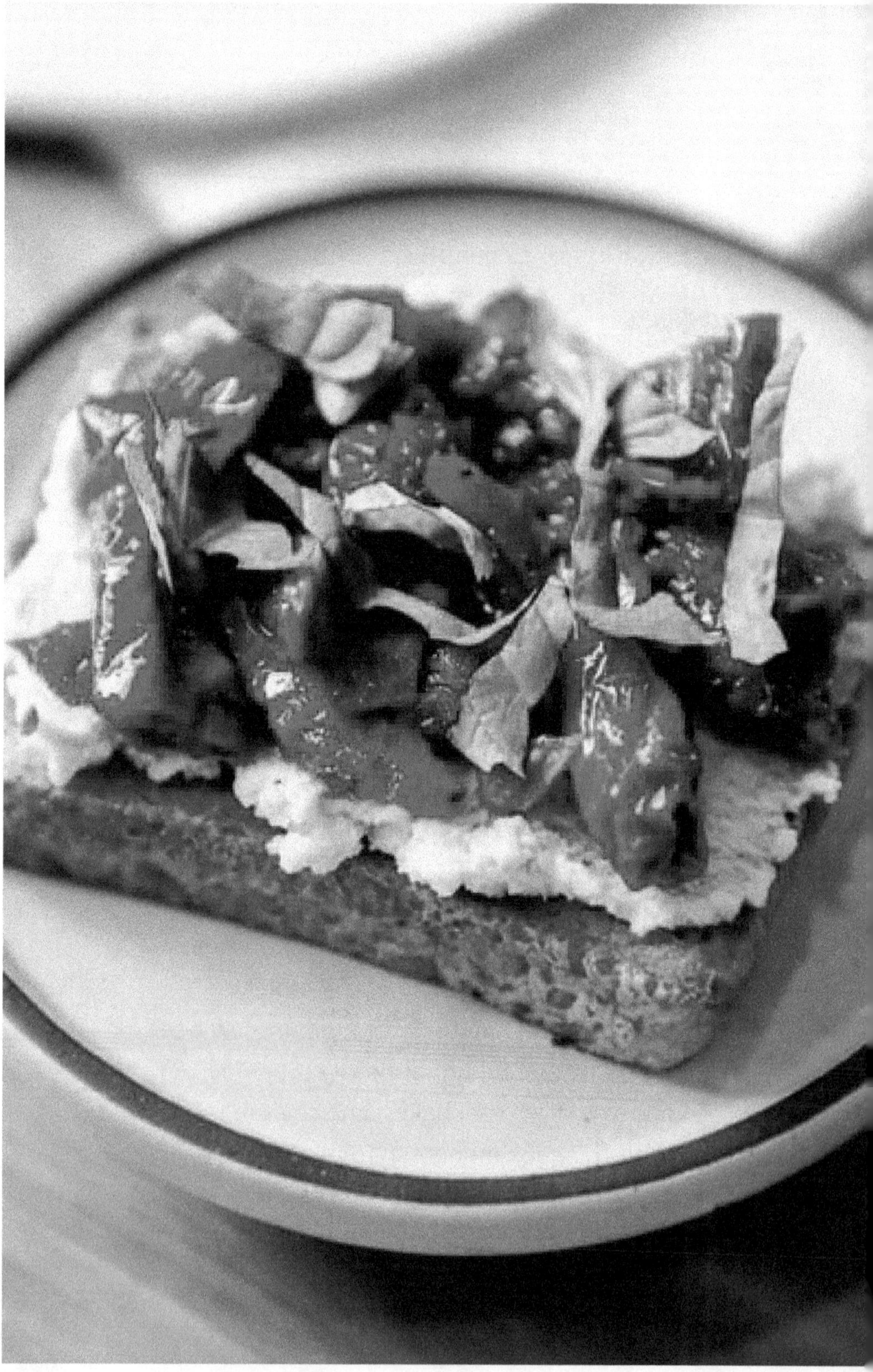

Spicy Chili Scramble

6 Servings

Preparation Time: 15 minutes

Ingredients

- 1 chili pepper, chopped
- 1½ tablespoons of butter
- 1½ cups water, for cooking
- 4 tomatoes
- 6 eggs
- 1 teaspoon of sea salt

Directions

- Add water into the saucepan and bring it to boil.
- Remove water from the heat and add tomatoes.
- Let the tomatoes stay in hot water for 2-3 minutes.
- After this, remove the tomatoes from the water and peel them.
- Place butter in the pan and melt it.
- Add chopped chili pepper and fry it for 3 minutes over medium heat.
- Then chop the peeled tomatoes and add them into the chili peppers.

- Cook the vegetables for 5 minutes over medium heat. Stir them from time to time.
- After this, add sea salt and crack, then eggs.
- Stir (scramble) the eggs well with the help of the fork and cook them for 3 minutes over medium heat.

Pear Oatmeal with Cinnamon

6 Servings

Preparation Time: 25 minutes

Ingredients

- 1½ tablespoons Splenda
- 1½ teaspoons butter
- 1 teaspoon ground cinnamon
- 2 egg, beaten
- 1½ cupsoatmeal
- 1 cup milk
- 1½ pears, chopped
- 1½ teaspoons vanilla extract

Directions

- In the big bowl, mix up together oatmeal, milk, egg, vanilla extract, Splendid, and ground cinnamon.
- Melt butter and add it to the oatmeal mixture.
- Then add chopped pear and stir it well.
- Transfer the oatmeal mixture to the casserole mold and flatten gently. Cover it with foil and secure edges.
- Bake the oatmeal for 25 minutes at 350°F.

LUNCH

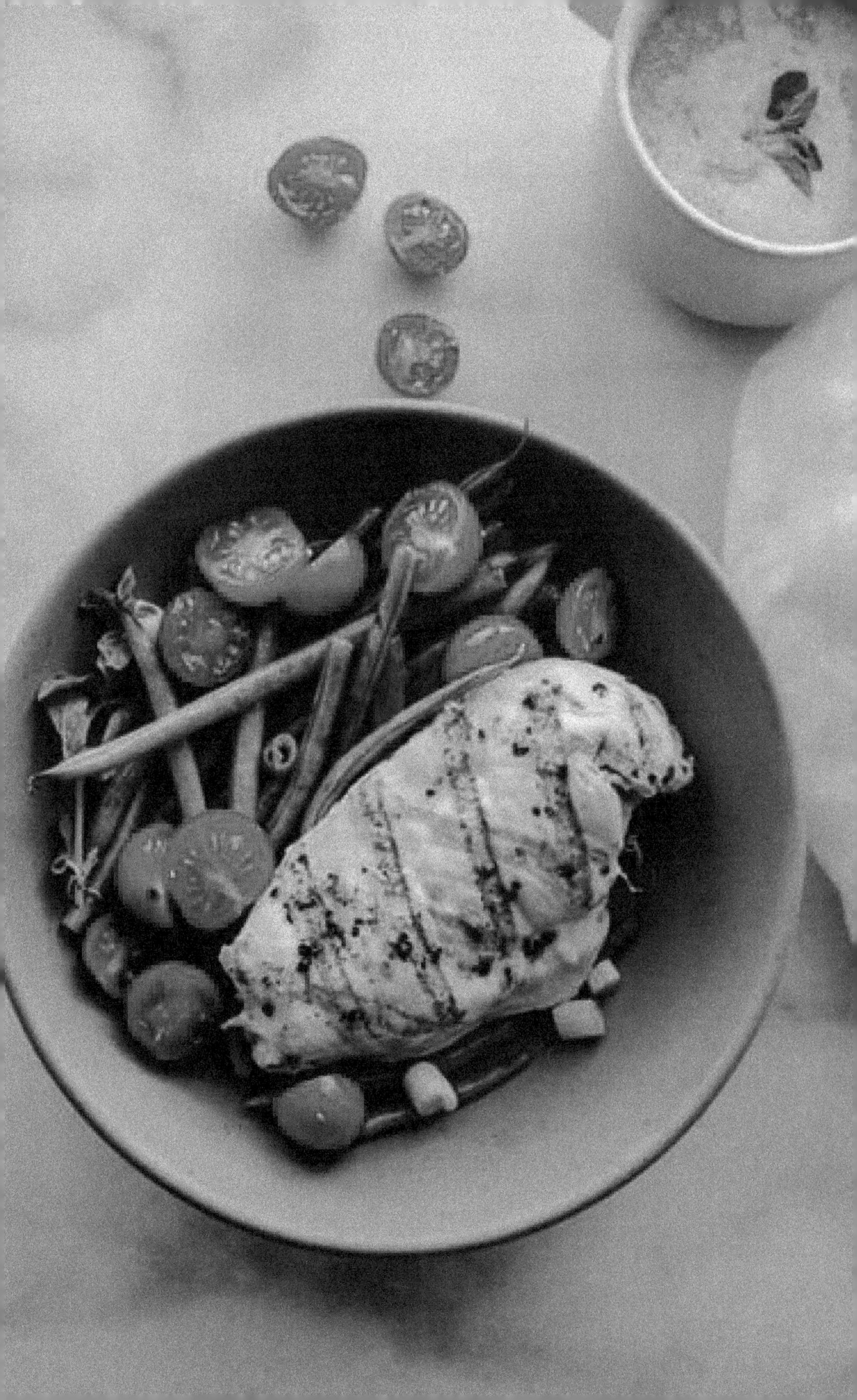

Tofu with Vegetable Scramble

2 Servings

Preparation Time: 20 minutes

Ingredients

- 1½ pinch of ground pepper.
- 1/3 cup canned chickpeas, rinsed.
- 1 cup pico de gallo or salsa.
- 1 cup shredded cheddar cheese, preferably sharp (1 oz.).
- 1½ dash hot sauce and chopped cilantro to taste.
- 1 ½ teaspoons extra-virgin olive oil.
- 5 ounces extra-firm tofu, drained, and cubed.
- 1½ cups chopped vegetables, such as zucchini, mushrooms, and onions.
- 1 teaspoon spice of choice, such as chili powder or ground cumin.

Directions

- Warm the oil in a large nonstick pan over medium-high heat. Add in the tofu, vegetables, spice, and pepper; cook, stirring often, until the vegetables are softened, 5 to 7 minutes.
- Add in chickpeas and pico de gallo and heat through for about 1 to 2 minutes.

- Remove from heat; gather the scramble into one section of the pan, top with Cheddar cheese, and let melt off the heat. Serve with hot sauce and cilantro.

Cauliflower Chickpea Curry with Cream

6 Servings

Preparation Time: 35 minutes

Ingredients

- 1½ cans of chickpeas 15 oz, drained and rinsed.
- 1½ cans dice tomatoes 15 oz.
- 1½ cans of coconut milk 14 oz.
- 2-3 tbsps fresh chopped cilantro.
- Salt and pepper, to taste.
- Rice, cauliflower rice, and/or naan for serving
- 2½ tbsps coconut oil.
- 1½ medium white onions diced.
- 3-4 garlic cloves minced.
- 1-inch fresh ginger peeled and grated.
- 2½ tbsps red curry paste.
- 1 ½large red bell pepper diced.
- 1 ½small cauliflower head chopped into small florets.

Directions

- Warm the large pan over medium-high heat and add in the coconut oil and onion.

- Cook for about 3-4 minutes, and then stir in garlic, ginger, red curry paste, and bell pepper. Continue to cook for about 2-3 minutes, stir it occasionally.
- Add in all the remaining ingredients: cauliflower florets, chickpeas, diced tomatoes, coconut milk, salt, and pepper.
- Reduce the heat and simmer until cauliflower is fork-tender and sauce thickens, about 10-12 minutes.
- Pour the curry into bowls and sprinkle with fresh chopped cilantro and serve hot.

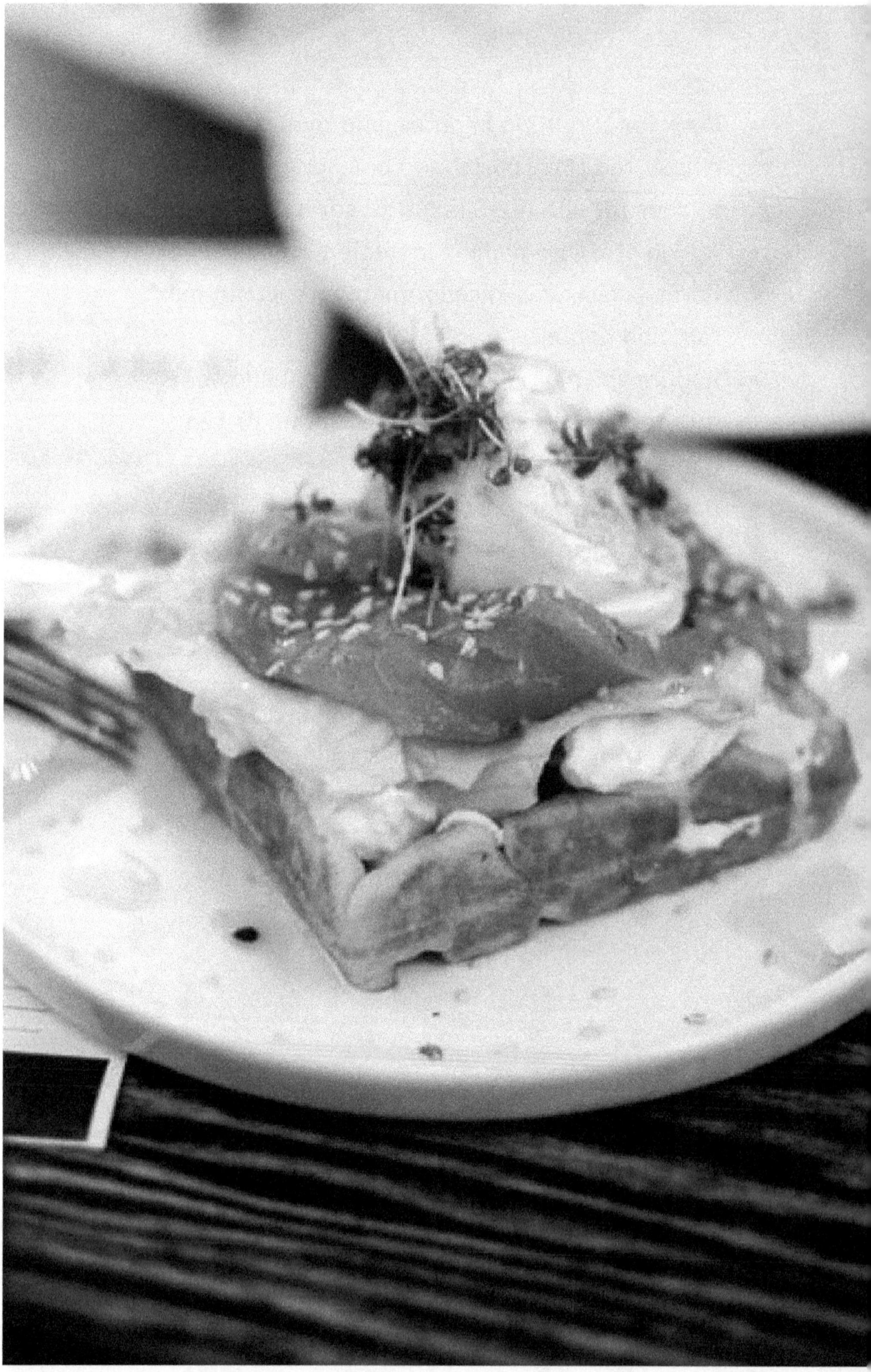

Cauliflower Risotto with Mushrooms

6 Servings

Preparation Time: 35 minutes

Ingredients

- 24 ounces fresh rice cauliflower.
- (8 cups) (such as eat smart).
- 1½ cups of tap water.
- 1 cup unsalted vegetable stock (such as imagine organic).
- 1 teaspoon kosher salt.
- 1 teaspoon black pepper.
- 2½ ounces parmesan cheese, finely shredded, divided (about 3/4 cup).

- 5½ tablespoons olive oil, divided.
- 6 ½ cups (10 oz.) Sliced fresh cremini mushrooms.
- 1 small (6 oz.) Yellow onion, finely chopped (about 1 cup).
- 2½ teaspoons finely chopped garlic (from 2 cloves).
- 2½ teaspoons fresh thyme leaves, plus leaves for garnish.
- 1 cup dry white wine.

Directions

- Warm 1 ½ tablespoons of the oil in a large pan over medium-high. Put half of the mushrooms, and cook until lightly browned, for about 5 minutes. Transfer the mushrooms to a plate. Repeat the process. Lower the heat to medium, and add in onion, garlic, thyme, and remaining 2 tablespoons oil; cook it, until softened, about 5 minutes. Add in wine; cook until the wine is absorbed for about 90 seconds. Add in the cauliflower, water, and stock. Cover and cook until cauliflower is crisp-tender, for about 10 to 12 minutes. Remove from heat.
- Pour 3 cups of the cauliflower mixture along with the remaining liquid in the pan into a blender. Secure the lid on the blender. Blend until smooth, about 15 seconds.
- Put the mixture in the pan on medium heat. Add in cauliflower puree, mushrooms, salt, pepper, and ¼ cup of cheese. Cook, until cheese is melted and mixture has a creamy consistency, for about 1 minute. Divide the risotto among 4 bowls; sprinkle evenly with remaining 1/2 cup cheese. Garnish with thyme leaves and serve immediately.

Portobello Mushrooms with Stuffed Spinach

6 Servings

Preparation Time: 40 minutes

Ingredients

- 1 (10 ounces) bag fresh spinach, chopped.
- 1 cup chopped pepperoni.
- 1 cup grated parmesan cheese.

- 5 large portobello mushroom caps, stems, and gills removed.
- 1½ tablespoons reduced-fat Italian salad dressing
- 2 eggs.
- 1½ cloves of garlic, minced.
- Salt and ground black pepper to taste.
- 1 cup shredded mozzarella cheese, divided.
- 3½ tablespoons seasoned bread crumbs, divided.

Directions

- Preheat oven to 350°F (175 degrees C).
- Apply Italian dressing on both sides of each Portobello mushroom cap. Place the mushroom on a baking sheet, gill sides up.
- Bake the mushrooms in the preheated oven until tender for about 12 minutes. Strain any juice that has formed in the mushrooms.

- Whisk the egg, garlic, salt, and black pepper together in a large bowl.
- Add in spinach, pepperoni, Parmesan cheese, 3 tablespoons mozzarella cheese, and 3 tablespoons of bread crumbs into the eggs until evenly mixed.
- Spread the spinach mixture over mushroom caps; sprinkle 1 tablespoon mozzarella cheese and 1 tablespoon bread crumbs on it. Return mushrooms to the oven.

Zucchini with Eggplant Gratin

8 Servings

Preparation Time: 55 minutes

Ingredients

- 1½ tbsps garlic powder.
- 1/3 cup freshly grated parmesan cheese or more.
- 2½ tbsps. olive oil.
- Sea salt and fresh ground black pepper.
- 2½ medium egg plants sliced into 1/4" slices.
- 2½ medium zucchini sliced into 1/4" slices.
- 1½ lbs. Vine ripe tomatoes sliced into 1/4" slices.
- 1 ½ tbsps Italian seasoning.

Directions

- Preheat the oven to 375⁰F and grease a baking dish with cooking spray.
- Add the eggplant, tomato, and zucchini slices in a large bowl. Drizzle with Italian seasoning, garlic powder, parmesan, and then spice with salt and pepper to taste.
- Shower some olive oil and mix to get all slices well coated.

- Place the sliced veggie into the prepared baking dish, making a spiral stack starting from the edge through the middle.
- Put the dish on a rack in the center of the oven and bake for about 40 minutes until vegetables are soft and the top is golden brown.

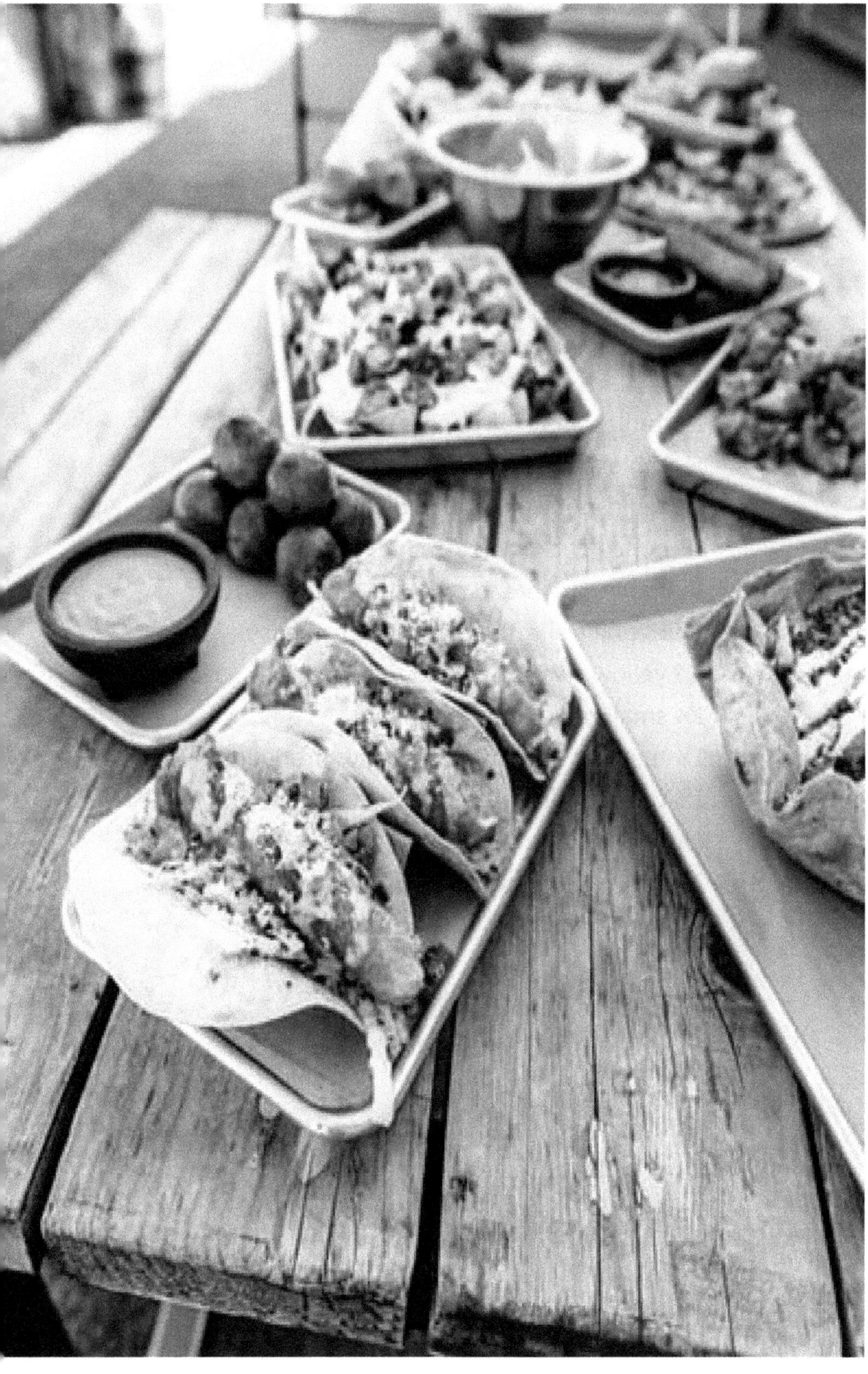

Portobello Mushrooms with Veggie Stuffing

6 Servings

Preparation Time: 32 minutes

Ingredients

- 2-3 tablespoons olive oil.
- 1½ tablespoons snipped fresh basil.
- 1½ tablespoons lemon juice.
- 15-ounce package fresh baby spinach.
- 1 cup fine dry bread crumbs.
- 1 cup finely shredded parmesan cheese.
- 1½ yellow sweet pepper cut in bite-size strips.
- 1½ small red onions, chopped.
- 1½ medium zucchinis, coarsely shredded.
- 1½ carrots coarsely shredded.
- 1½ celeries thinly sliced.
- 2½ cloves of garlic, minced.
- 4 inches portobello mushroom caps, stems removed.
- 4 Slices Provolone Cheese.

Directions

- Preheat the oven to 425°F. Line a baking pan with foil. In a 12-inch pan, cook and add in sweet pepper, onion, zucchini, carrot, celery, and garlic in hot oil over medium-high heat for 4 minutes. Add in basil, parsley, lemon juice, ¼ teaspoon of each salt, and ground black pepper. Top with spinach; cover. Cook for 2 minutes or until spinach is wilted. Remove from heat. Add crumbs and half of the Parmesan cheese into spinach mixture; set aside.

- Remove the gills from mushrooms. Place the mushrooms, stemmed side up, on the prepared pan. Top each with a slice of provolone cheese. Divide the spinach mixture among mushroom caps. Bake for 15 minutes. Top with the remaining parmesan. Bake for 2 minutes more. Makes 4 servings.

Beef Meatballs with Marinara Sauce and Parsley

6 Servings

Preparation Time: 45 minutes

Ingredients

- 1 egg, beaten
- 1½ pounds ground beef
- 2 cloves of garlic, minced
- 1 tbsp olive oil
- 1 cup breadcrumbs
- ½ cup parmesan cheese, grated
- ½ cup milk
- 6 cups marinara sauce
- Chopped parsley to garnish
- Salt and black pepper to taste

Directions

- Line a baking pan with foil and oil it with cooking spray. Set aside.

- Mix the milk and breadcrumbs in a bowl.

- Add the ground beef, garlic, Parmesan cheese, egg, salt, and black pepper, until combined.

- Make the balls of the mixture and place them in the prepared pan.

- Preheat the oven to 350ºF. Bake the meatballs for 20 minutes.

- Pour the marinara sauce into a saucepan and bring to a simmer, stirring for about 10 minutes.

- Arrange the meatballs on a platter and spoon the marinara sauce on top.

- Sprinkle with chopped parsley to serve.

Baked Fish with Parmesan Cheese Topping

4 Servings

Preparation Time: 40 minutes

Ingredients

- 1 tbsp olive oil
- ½ pound tilapia fillets, cubed
- 1 cup tomato sauce
- ½ pound cod, cubed
- ¼ cup Parmesan cheese, grated
- 1 broccoli, cut into florets
- Parmesan cheese, grated for topping
- Sea salt and black pepper to taste

Directions

- Grease a baking dish with cooking spray.

- Place the fish and broccoli in oil and sprinkle with salt and black pepper. Then Spread in the greased dish.

- Mix the tomato sauce with Parmesan cheese, pour and smear the cream over the fish, and sprinkle with some more Parmesan.

- Bake for 25 minutes in the oven at 400ºF, take the dish out.

- Finally, serve into plates.

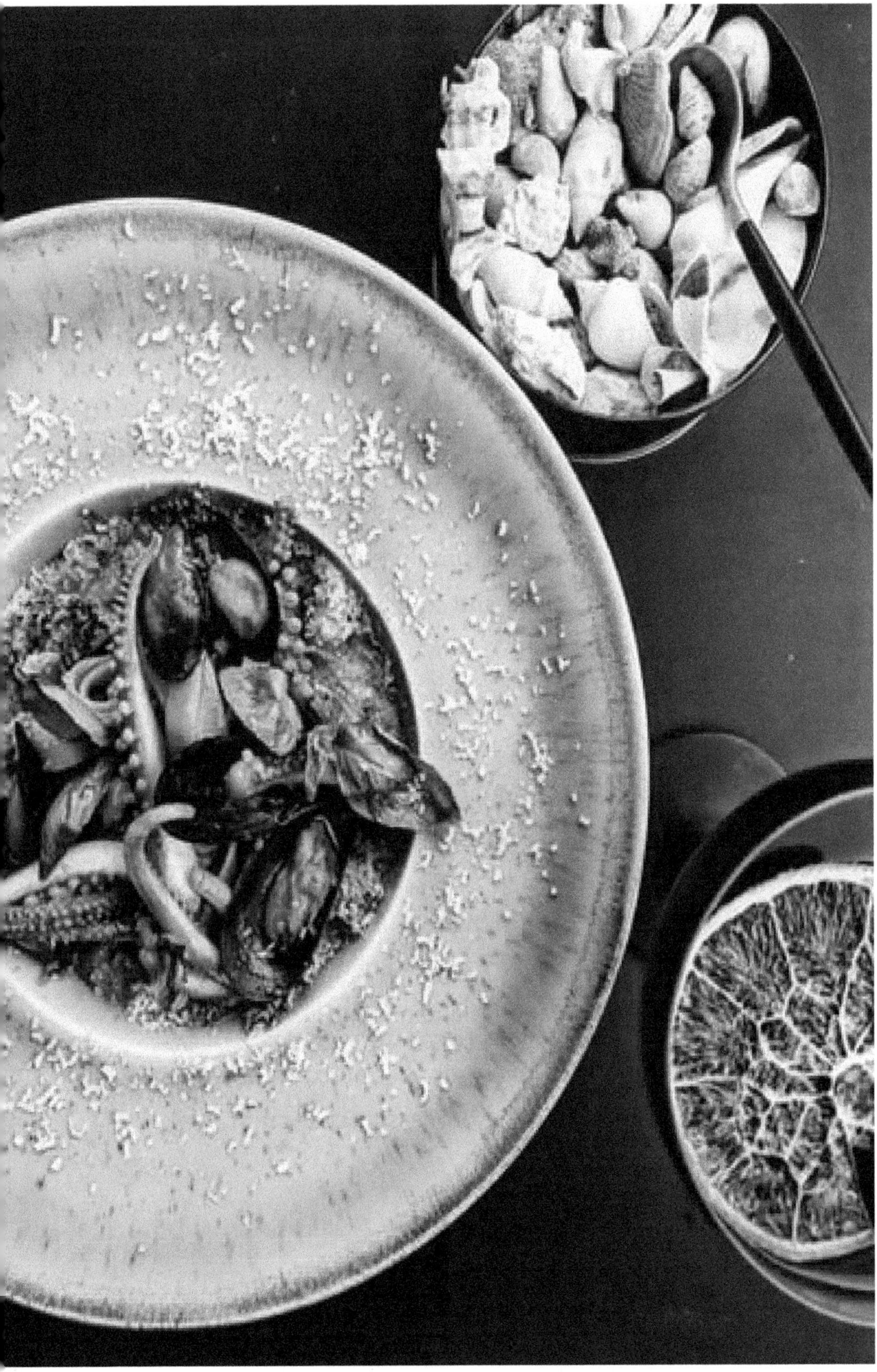

Feta Cheese & Zucchini Gratin

6 Servings

Preparation Time: 65 minutes

Ingredients

- 2 tbsps olive oil
- 2 green bell peppers, seeded and sliced
- 12 oz feta cheese, crumbled
- 4 zucchinis, sliced and squeezed
- ¼ tsp cornstarch
- ½ cup milk
- ⅓ cup mozzarella cheese for topping
- Salt and black pepper to taste

Directions

- On a baking dish, grease it with a cooking spray and make a layer of zucchini and bell peppers in the dish overlapping one on another.

- Sprinkle some black pepper and some feta cheese. Repeat the layering process a second time.

- Mix the olive oil, cornstarch, and milk in a microwave dish for 2 minutes, stir to mix completely, and spread over the vegetables.

- Spread over mozzarella cheese. Bake the gratin for 45 minutes to be golden brown on top.

- Cut out slices and serve with salad.

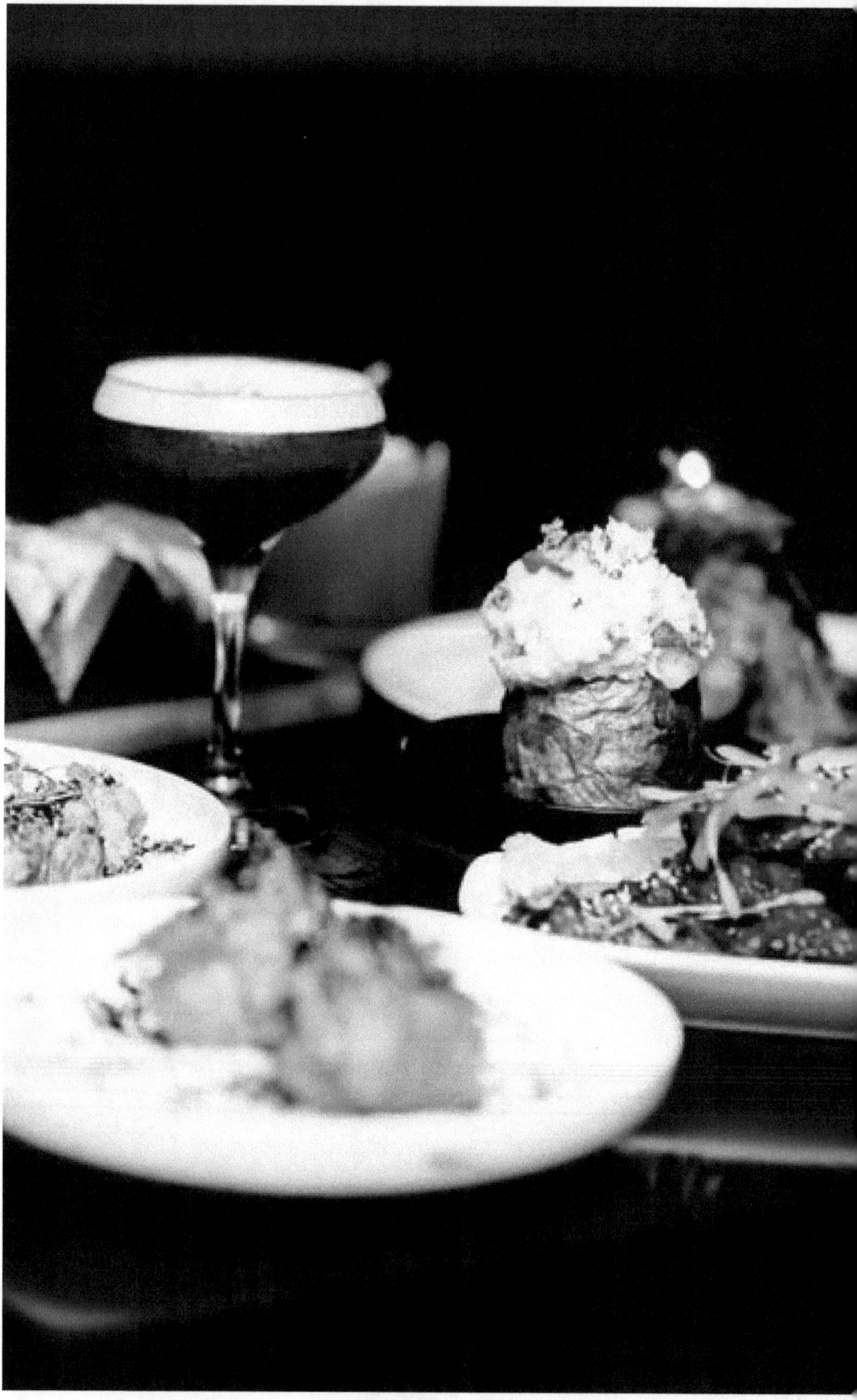

BRUNCH

Honey-roasted Cherry with Ricotta Tartine

6 Servings

Preparation Time: 15 minutes

Ingredients

- 1½ tablespoons lemon juice
- 1½ tablespoons honey, plus more for serving
- 1½ cups ricotta cheese, part-skim
- Pinch of flaky sea salt, such as Maldon
- Pinch of salt
- 6 slices (1/2 inch thick) artisan bread, whole-grain
- 3 cups fresh cherries, pitted
- 3 teaspoons extra-virgin olive oil
- 1 cup slivered almonds, toasted
- 1½ teaspoons lemon zest
- 1½ teaspoons fresh thyme

Directions:

- Preheat oven to 400°F. Line a rimmed baking sheet with parchment paper; set aside.
- In a mixing bowl, toss the cherries with honey, oil, lemon juice, and salt. Transfer into the pan. Roast for about 15 minutes, shaking the pan once or twice during roasting until the cherries are very soft and warm.

- Toast the bread. Top with the cheese, cherries, thyme, lemon zest, almonds, and season with sea salt. If desired, drizzle more honey.

Cheesy Eggs Mix

4 Servings

Preparation Time: 5 min

Ingredients

- 1 teaspoon salt
- 1½ teaspoons butter
- 1½ teaspoons fresh parsley, chopped
- 6 eggs, beaten
- 1 teaspoon ground black pepper
- 3 oz Feta, scrambled

Directions:

- Melt butter in the skillet and add beaten eggs.
- Then add parsley, salt, and scrambled eggs. Cook the eggs for 1 minute over high heat.
- Add ground black pepper and scramble eggs with the help of the fork.
- Cook the eggs for 3 minutes over medium-high heat.

Spicy Chili Avocado Scramble

6 Servings

Preparation Time: 15 minutes

Ingredients

- 1 teaspoon chili flakes
- 1½ oz Cheddar cheese, shredded
- 1 teaspoon salt
- 1½ tablespoons fresh parsley
- 6 eggs, beaten
- 1 white onion, diced
- 1 tablespoon avocado oil
- 1 avocado, finely chopped

Directions:

- Pour avocado oil in the skillet and bring it to boil.
- Then add diced onion and roast it until it is light brown.
- Meanwhile, mix up together chili flakes, beaten eggs, and salt.
- Pour the egg mixture over the cooked onion and cook the mixture for 1 minute over medium heat.
- After this, scramble the eggs well with the help of the fork or spatula. Cook the eggs until they are solid but soft.

- After this, add chopped avocado and shredded cheese.
- Stir the scramble well and transfer in the serving plates. Sprinkle the meal with fresh parsley.

Baked Egg and Pepper

6 Servings

Preparation Time: 28 minutes

Ingredients

- 1½ teaspoons paprika
- 1½ tablespoons fresh cilantro, chopped
- 1½ garlic clove, diced
- 1½ teaspoons butter, softened
- 1 teaspoon chili flakes
- 3 eggs, beaten
- 1½ red bell peppers, chopped
- 1½ chili peppers, chopped
- 1 red onion, diced
- 1½ teaspoons canola oil
- 1 teaspoon salt

Directions

- Brush the casserole mold with canola oil and pour beaten eggs inside.
- After this, toss the butter in the skillet and melt it over medium heat.
- Add chili pepper and red bell pepper.
- After this, add red onion and cook the vegetables for 7-8 minutes over medium heat. Stir them from time to time.

- Transfer the vegetables into the casserole mold.
- Add salt, paprika, cilantro, diced garlic, and chili flakes. Stir gently with the help of a spatula to get a homogenous mixture.
- Bake the casserole for 20 minutes at 355F in the oven.
- Then chill the meal well and cut into servings. Transfer the casserole into the serving plates with the help of the spatula.

Easy Feta Spinach Balls

10 Servings

Preparation Time: 30 minutes

Ingredients

- 3 eggs, beaten
- 1 cup feta cheese, crumbled
- 1 tsp nutmeg
- 1½ cups flour
- 1 tsp black pepper
- 4 tbsps melted butter
- 3 tbsps butter, melted
- 1½ tbsps of onion powder
- 1 cup Parmesan cheese, grated
- 10 oz spinach

Directions

- Preheat the oven to 350ºF.
- Put all ingredients in a food processor. Blend until smooth.
- Put in the freezer for about 10 minutes.
- Now make balls out of the mixture and arrange them on a lined baking sheet.
- Bake for 10-12 minutes.

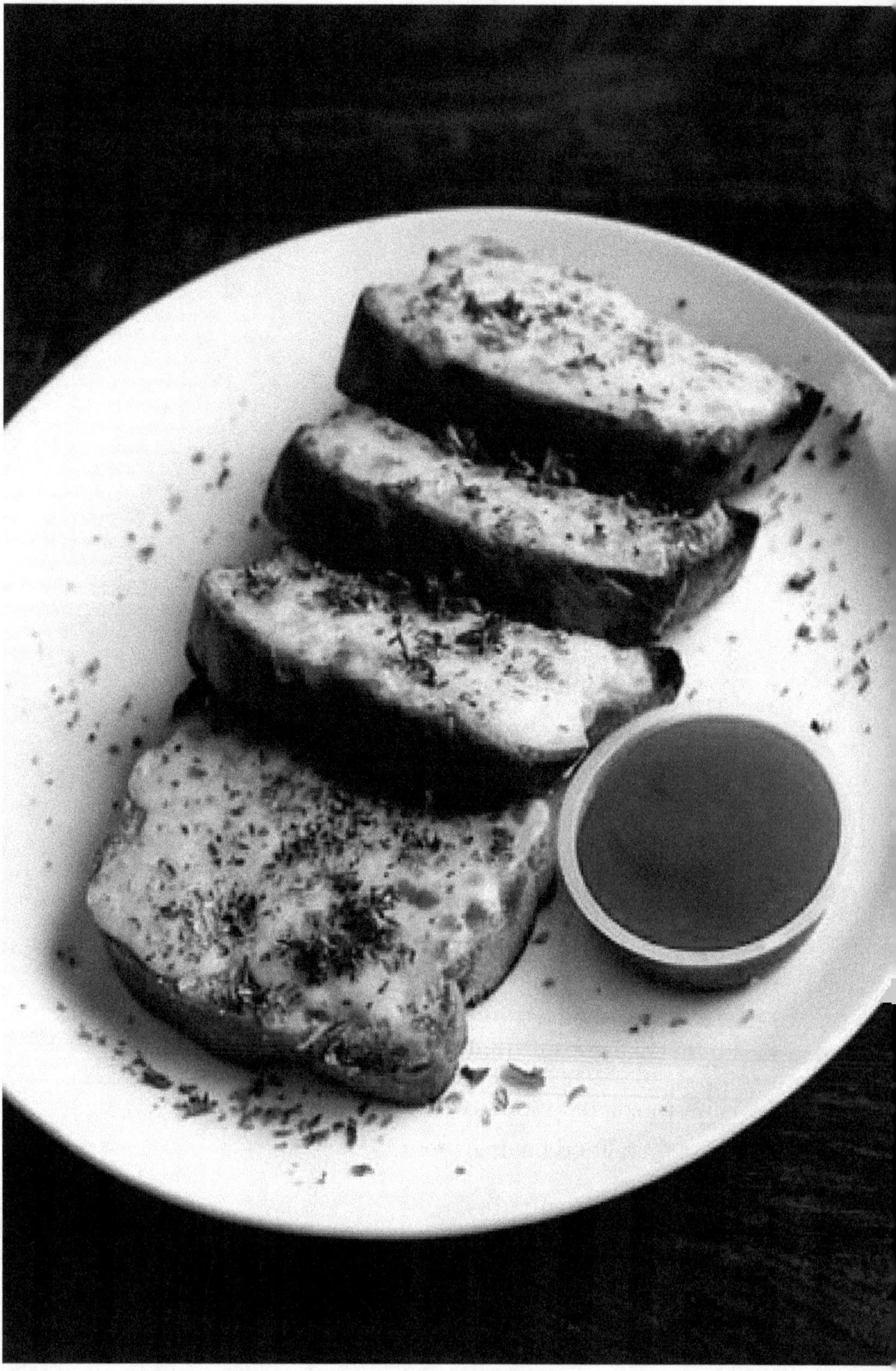

Stuffed Avocado with Spicy Tuna

6 Servings

Preparation Time: 20 minutes

Ingredients

- 3 tbsps chives, chopped
- 3 avocados, halved and pitted
- 3 tbsps capers
- 6 oz mozzarella cheese, grated
- 3 oz canned tuna, flaked
- 1 cup curly endive, chopped
- Salt and black pepper, to taste

Directions

- Place the avocado halves in an ovenproof dish.

- Combine the chives, black pepper, salt, capers, and tuna.

- Stuff the tuna mixture in the avocado halves. Top with grated cheese.

- Bake in the oven for 15 minutes at 360ºF or until the top is golden brown.

Mascarpone Cheese & Carrot Mousse

8 Servings

Preparation Time: 15 min + cooling time

Ingredients

- 4 eggs
- 2 cups half & half
- 1 cup sugar
- 1 cup mascarpone
- 1 tsp ground cloves
- 2 cups canned carrots
- 1 tsp grated nutmeg
- 1 tsp ground cinnamon
- A pinch of salt

Directions

- Mix sugar, mascarpone, and half & half, and boil in a saucepan over medium heat.

- Whisk the eggs; slowly place in ½ of the hot cream mixture to the beaten eggs.

- Spread the mixture back to the pan.

- Cook for about 2 to 4 minutes, until thick. Turn off the heat; add in the carrots, cinnamon, salt, nutmeg, and cloves.

- Blend with a blender and split the mixture among serving plates, and refrigerate it.

Nuts and Endive with Salsa Roquefort

6 Servings

Preparation Time: 15 min + cooling time

Ingredients

- 3 cups heavy cream
- 3 endive heads, leaves separated
- 1 tsp nutmeg
- 6 oz Roquefort cheese, crumbled
- 1 cup toasted pine nuts
- Salt and black pepper to taste

Directions

- Warm heavy cream in a saucepan over medium heat. Add in the Roquefort cheese, nutmeg, salt, and pepper and mix well.

- Transfer it to a bowl and whisk with a mixer until smooth. Let it cool.

- Place the endive leaves on a serving plate.

- Spoon the Roquefort mixture into the leaves and top with the pine nuts to serve.

DINNER

72

Instant Pot Chicken and Broccoli

6 Servings

Preparation Time: 20 minutes

Ingredients

- 1½ cups unsalted walnuts
- 1½ pounds of chicken breasts, cut into strips
- 1½ tsps sugar
- 4½ tbsps olive oil
- 3 tsps balsamic vinegar
- 3 cups broccoli florets
- 3 tsps cornstarch
- 1½ lemon, juiced
- Pepper to taste
- 1½ white onion, thinly sliced

Directions

- Mix the vinegar, lemon juice, sugar, and cornstarch in a bowl and set aside.

- Heat the oil in a pan and fry the walnuts for about 2 minutes until golden brown.

- Place the walnuts on a paper towel-lined plate.

- Sauté the onion in the same oil for 4 minutes until soft and browned, then add the walnuts.

- Now add the chicken to the pan and cook for more 4 minutes also include the broccoli and pepper with the chicken.

- Pour the soy sauce mixture into it.

- Cook the sauce for approximately 4 minutes and add in the walnuts and onion.

- Cook for 1 minute, and then turn the heat off.

- Serve the chicken stir-fry with a green salad.

Gorgonzola with Bell Peppers

6 Servings

Preparation Time: 45 minutes

Ingredients

- 2 cups tomatoes, pureed
- 3 tbspsolive oil
- 8 oz gorgonzola cheese, crumbled
- 1 tsp chili pepper
- 6 red bell peppers, blanched
- 8 oz cottage cheese
- 1 cup breadcrumbs
- 1 oregano
- 3 cloves garlic, smashed
- 1½ tsps dried basil
- Salt and black pepper, to taste

Directions

- Preheat oven to 360°F.

- Lightly brush the sides and bottom of a Crockpot dish with olive oil.

- Mix garlic, cottage cheese, breadcrumbs, and gorgonzola cheese in a bowl.

- Stuff the peppers and add in the Crockpot dish.

- Mix the tomato puree with oregano, salt, cayenne pepper, black pepper, and basil.

- Spread the tomato mixture over stuffed peppers and cover the dish with foil.

- Bake for 40 minutes until the peppers are tender.

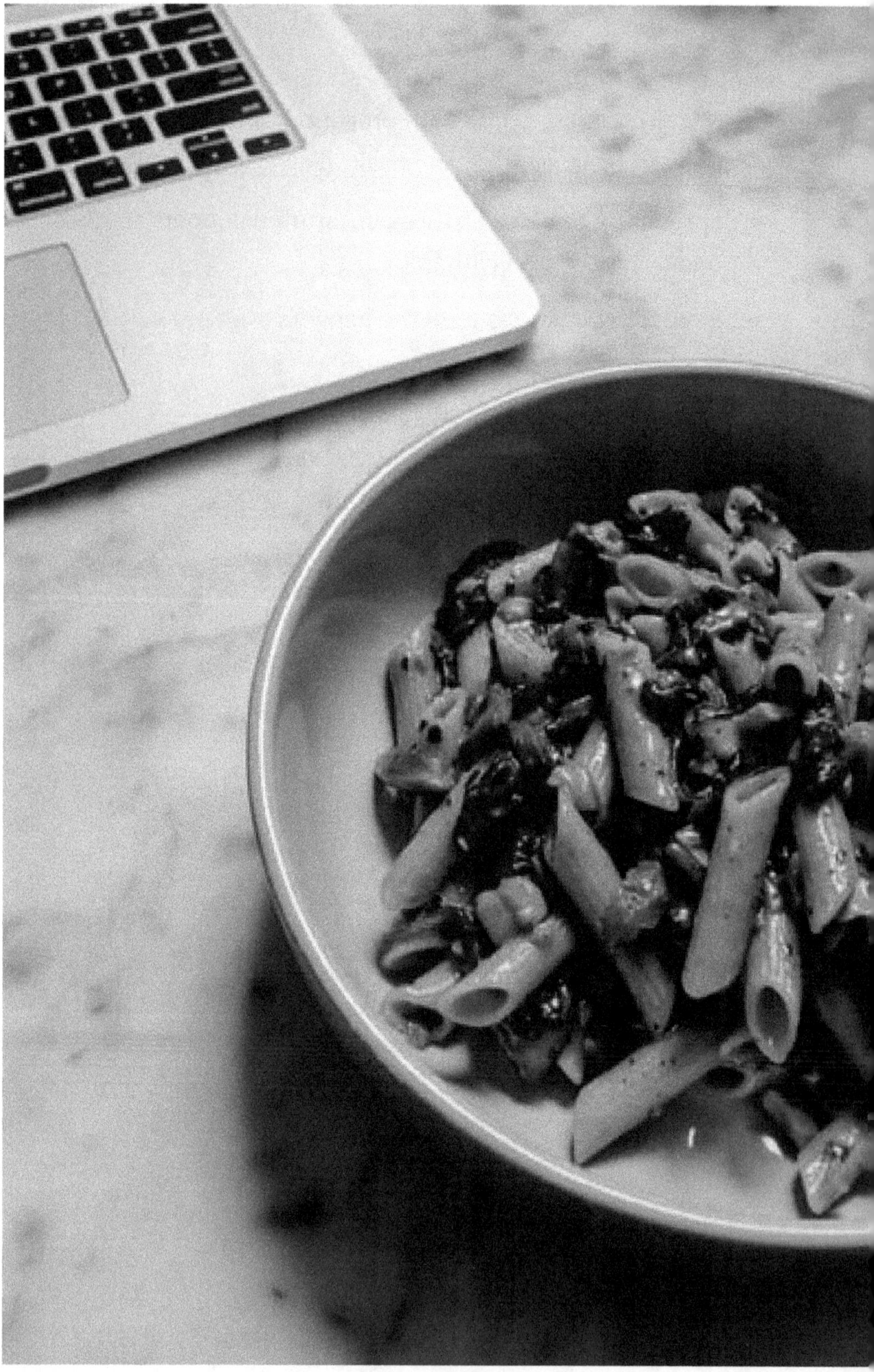

Crispy Chicken Wings with Parmesan & Yogurt Sauce

8 Servings

Preparation Time: 25 minutes

Ingredients

Wings
- Cooking spray
- 2½ pounds chicken wings
- 1 cup Hot sauce
- 1 cup olive oil
- 1 cup Parmesan cheese, grated
- Salt and black pepper to taste

Yogurt Sauce
- 1½ cups plain yogurt
- Salt and black pepper to taste
- 1 ½ tsps fresh lemon juice

Directions
- Preheat oven to 400⁰F. And flavor the wings with salt and pepper.
- Put the wings on a baking sheet and brush with oil.
- Bake for 20 minutes until golden brown.

- Mix the yogurt, lemon juice, salt, and black pepper in a bowl.

- Mix the olive oil, hot sauce, and parmesan in a bowl. Mix up the chicken in the sauce to evenly coat and plate.

- Serve with yogurt dipping sauce.

Stuffed Chicken Breasts with tasty Basil Tomato Sauce

8 Servings

Preparation Time: 45 minutes

Ingredients

- 2 pounds chicken breasts
- 1 cup cottage cheese
- 1 cup yogurt
- 1½ tbsps. olive oil
- 8 mozzarella slices
- ¼ cup mozzarella, shredded
- 2½ cups kale, chopped
- 1½ cups tomato basil sauce

Directions

- Mix up the cottage cheese, yogurt, shredded mozzarella, and put in the microwave.
- Cut the chicken with the knife horizontally.
- Stuff with the filling. Brush the chicken with olive oil.
- Place on a lined baking dish and put it in the oven. Bake the chicken in the oven for about 25 minutes at 400°F.

- Add the tomato basil sauce over and top with mozzarella slices.

- Return to oven and cook for more 5 minutes until the cheese melts.

Chicken Goujons

4 Servings

Preparation Time: 25 minutes

Ingredients

- 2 eggs, beaten
- 1 pound chicken breasts, cubed
- 1 cup olive oil
- 1 cup flour
- 4 tbsps garlic powder
- Salt and black pepper to taste

Directions

- Mix together salt, garlic powder, flour, and black pepper in a bowl.

- Chink the egg and beat the egg, then add the chicken cubes into the flour mixture.

- On medium heat, set the pan and warm olive oil, add the chicken nuggets, and cook for approximately 6 minutes on each side.

- Put on paper towels, drain the excess grease and serve.

Grilled Asparagus with Pancetta Wrapped Chicken

6 Servings

Preparation Time: 48 minutes

Ingredients

- 6 tbsps olive oil
- 1½ pounds of chicken breasts, boneless
- 1½ lbs asparagus spears
- 12 pancetta slices
- 3 tbsps fresh lemon juice
- Pecorino cheese for topping
- Salt and black pepper to taste

Directions

- Add salt and black pepper on chicken breasts, and wrap 2 pancetta slices around each chicken breast.

- Preheat oven to 370°F.

- Fix up on a baking sheet that is lined with parchment paper, trickle with 2 tbsps of olive oil and bake for 25-30 minutes until pancetta is brown and crispy.

- Preheat your grill on high heat.

- Brush the asparagus spears with olive oil and season with salt.

- Grill for approximately 8-10 minutes, frequently turning until slightly charred.

- Add to a plate and drizzle with lemon juice.

- Shred over Pecorino so that it melts a little with the hot asparagus and forms a cheesy dressing.

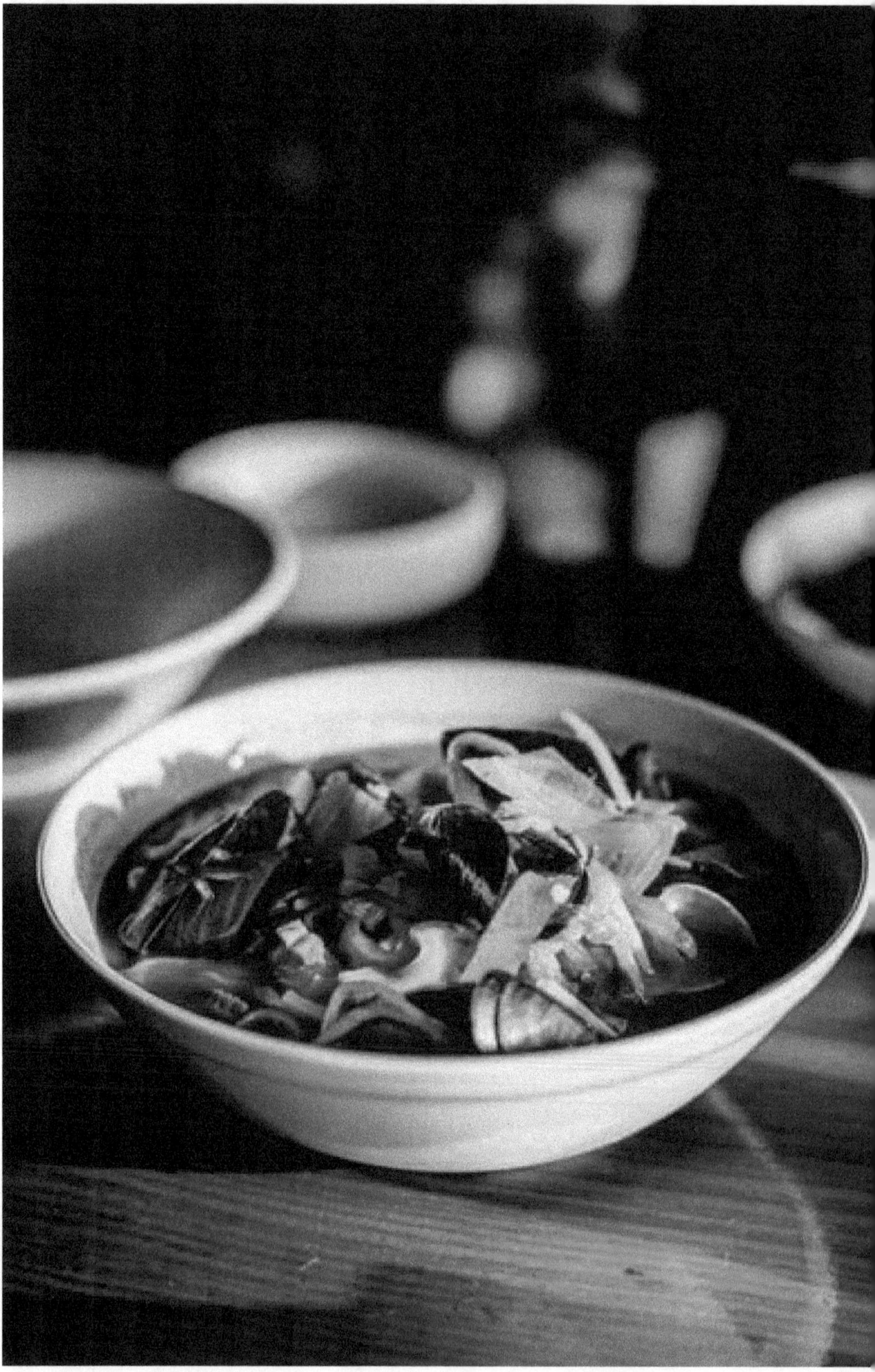

Cheesy Turkey with Hot Red Sauce

6 Servings

Preparation Time: 20 minutes

Ingredients

- 1½ tbsps. fresh parsley, chopped
- 10 oz mozzarella cheese, shredded
- 2½ tbsps. of tomato paste
- 1½ tbsps. olive oil
- ¼ cup chicken broth
- 1½ pounds turkey breasts, sliced
- 2½ garlic cloves, minced
- 1 cup tomato sauce

Directions

- Set a pan on medium heat with oil; add garlic and turkey and fry for about 4 minutes and set aside.

- Mix the broth, tomato paste, and tomato sauce and cook it until the puree thickened.

- Put the turkey in the pan; spread grated cheese over.

- Put it on rest for 5 minutes and cover until the cheese melts.

- Sprinkle the parsley and serve.

Turkey Meatballs

6 Servings

Preparation Time: 15 minutes

Ingredients

- 3 tbsps olive oil
- 1½ lbs ground turkey
- 1 cup flour
- 9 sun-dried tomatoes, chopped
- Salt and black pepper to taste
- 12 fresh basil leaves, chopped
- 2 eggs
- 1 cup provolone cheese, shredded
- 1½ tbsps dijon mustard
- 1 tsp Italian seasoning

Directions

- In a bowl, place all the ingredients except oil.
- Assemble with your hands until the ingredients merged.
- Make 16 meatballs with the mixture.
- Warm olive oil in a pan over medium heat.
- Cook the meatballs for about 3 minutes per each side.
- Serve with the zucchini spaghetti and tomato sauce.

DESSERT

Coconut with Risotto Pudding

6 Servings

Preparation Time: 20 minutes

Ingredients

- Three quarters cup rice
- Half cup shredded coconut
- 1 tsp lemon juice
- Half tsp vanilla
- Oz can coconut milk
- 1/4 cup maple syrup
- 1 Half cups water

Directions:

- Add all ingredients into the instant pot and mix well.
- Seal pot with lid and cook on high for 20 minutes.
- Once done, allow to release pressure naturally for 10 minutes, then release remaining using quick release. Remove lid.
- Keeps blending pudding mixture using an immersion keep blending er until smooth.
- Serve and enjoy.

Muesli Parfaits

4 Servings

Preparation Time: 10 minutes

Ingredients

- 4 cups Greek yogurt
- 1 cup whole wheat muesli
- 2 cups fresh berries of your choice

Directions:

- Layer the four glasses with Greek yogurt at the bottom, muesli on top, and berries.
- Repeat the layers until the glass is full.
- Place in the fridge for around 2 hours to chill.

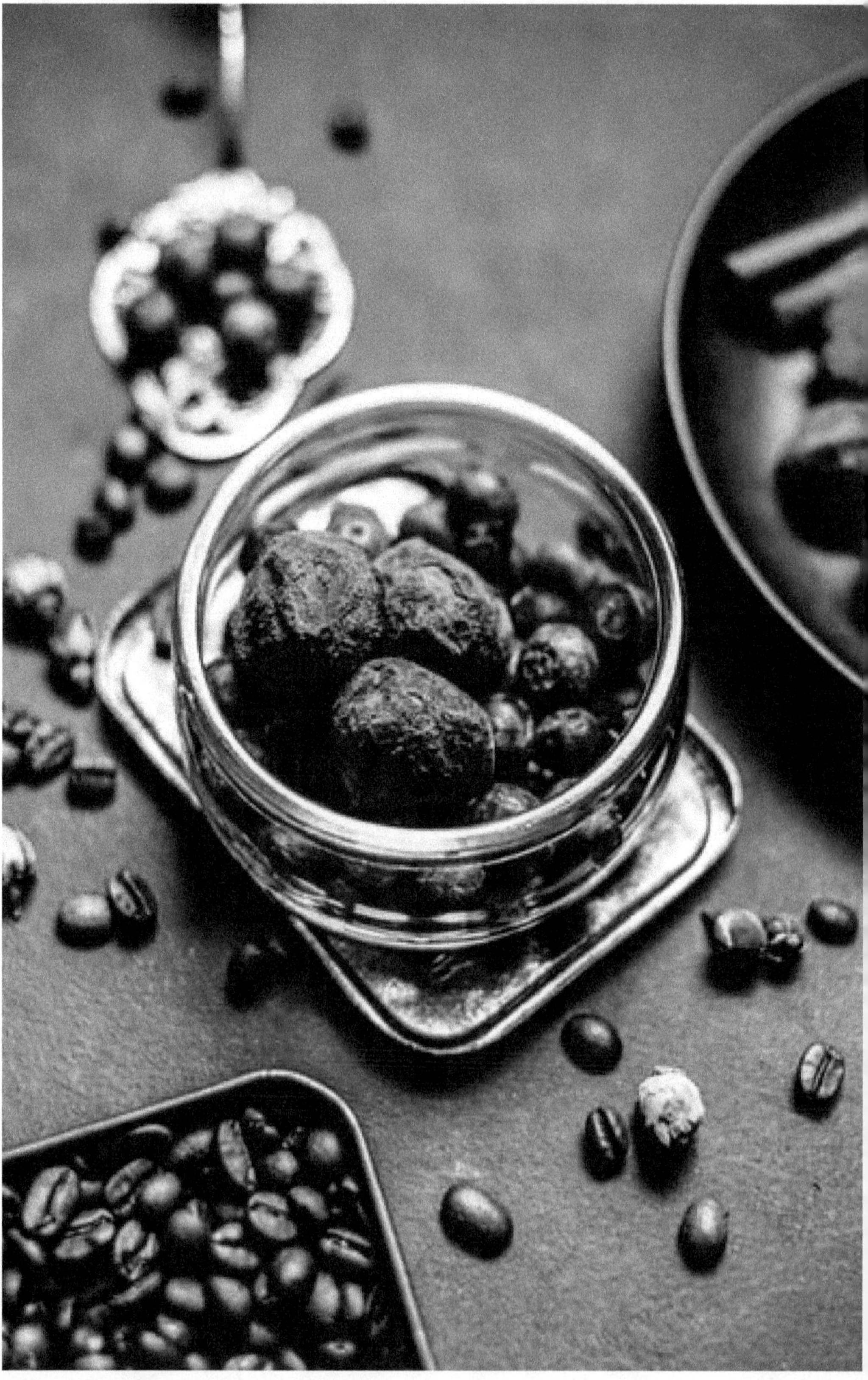

Seasonal Fruit Tart

1 Serving

Preparation Time: 15 minutes

Ingredients

- Half cups all-purpose flour
- Half tsp salt.
- 2 tablespoons sugar
- 1 cup cold butter
- Half cup shortening.
- 5 tablespoons of ice water
- 2 cups Ashta Custard
- Strawberries, sliced.
- 2 kiwis peeled and sliced.
- 1 cup blueberries
- 1 cup peach or apricot jam
- 3 tablespoons of water

Directions:

- In a food processor fitted with a chopping blade, pulse 2 cups all-purpose flour, salt, and sugar 5 times.
- Add butter and shortening and Keep blending for 1 minute or until mixture is crumbly.
- Transfer mixture to a medium bowl.

- Add ice water to the batter and mix just until combined.
- Place dough on a piece of plastic wrap, form into a flat disc and refrigerate for 20 minutes.
- Preheat the oven to 450ºF.
- Dust your workspace with flour, and using a rolling pin, roll out dough to 1/8-inch thickness.
- Place rolled-out dough into a 9-inch tart pan, press to mold into the pan, and cut off excess dough. Bake for 13 minutes.
- Let the tart cool for 10 minutes.
- Place tart shell on a serving dish, and fill with Ashta Custard.
- Arrange strawberry slices, kiwi slices, and blueberries on top of the tart.
- In a small saucepan over medium heat, heat peach jam and water, mixing, for 2 minutes.
- Using a pastry brush, brush the top of the fruit and tart with warmed jam.
- Serve chilled and store in the refrigerator.

Green Tea Vanilla Cream

4 Servings

Preparation Time: 5 minutes

Ingredients

- 14 ounces almond milk, hot
- 2 tbsps green tea powder
- 14 ounces heavy cream
- 3 tbsps stevia
- 1 tsp. vanilla extract
- 1 tsp. gelatin powder

Directions:

- In a bowl, combine the almond milk with the green tea powder and the rest of the ingredients, whisk well, cool down.
- Divide into cups and keep in the fridge for 2 hours before serving.

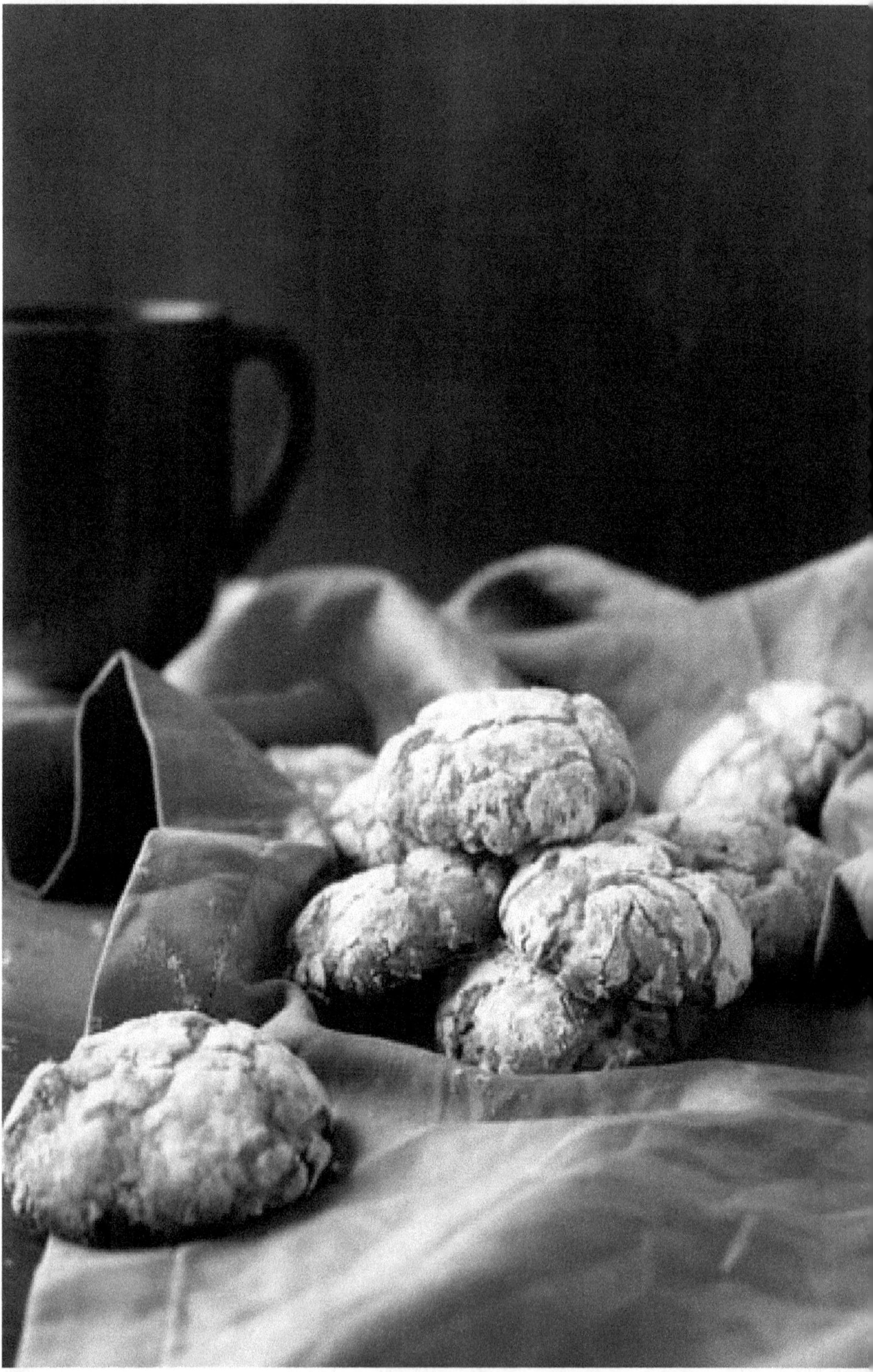

Sweet Semolina Pie

6 Servings

Preparation Time: 60 minutes

Ingredients

- Half cup milk.
- 3 tbsps. semolina
- Half cup butter, softened.
- 8 Phyllo sheets
- 2 eggs, beaten.
- 3 tbsps. Erythritol
- 1 tsp. lemon rind
- 1 tablespoon lemon juice
- 1 tsp. vanilla extract
- 2 tbsps. liquid honey
- 1 tsp. ground cinnamon
- ¼ cup of water

Directions:

- Melt half part of all butter.
- Then brush the casserole glass mold with the butter and place 1 Phyllo sheet inside.
- Brush the phyllo sheet with butter and cover it with a second Phyllo sheet.

- Make the dessert filling: heat up milk and add semolina.
- Mix it carefully.
- After this, add the remaining softened butter, Erythritol, and vanilla extract.
- Bring the mixture to boil and simmer it for 2 minutes.
- Remove it from the heat and cool to room temperature.
- Then add beaten eggs and mix up well.
- Transfer the semolina mixture in the mold over the Phyllo sheets, flatten it if needed.
- Then cover the semolina mixture with remaining Phyllo sheets and brush with remaining melted butter.
- Cut the dessert on the bars.
- Bake galaktoboureko for 1 hour at 365F.
- Then make the syrup: bring to boil lemon juice, honey, and water and remove the liquid from the heat.
- Transfer the syrup over the hot dessert and let it chill well.

Apple with Vanilla Compote

6 Servings

Preparation Time: 15 minutes

Ingredients

- 3 cups apples cored and cubed.
- 1 tsp vanilla
- Three quarters cup coconut sugar
- 1 cup of water
- 2 tbsps fresh lime juice

Directions:

- Add all ingredients into the inner pot of instant pot and mix well.
- Seal pot with lid and cook on high for 15 minutes.
- Once done, allow to release pressure naturally for 10 minutes, then release remaining using quick release. Remove lid.
- Mix and serve.

Cold Lemon Bites

4 Servings

Preparation Time: 5 minutes

Ingredients

- 1 cup avocado oil+ a drizzle
- 2 bananas peeled and chopped.
- 1 tablespoon honey
- ¼ cup lemon juice
- A pinch of lemon zest, grated.

Directions:

- In your food processor, mix the bananas with the rest of the ingredients.
- Pulse well and spread on the bottom of a pan greased with a drizzle of oil.
- Introduce in the fridge for 30 minutes, slice into squares and serve.

Coconut Cream with mint

2 Servings

Preparation Time: 5 minutes

Ingredients

- 1 banana, peeled.
- 2 cups coconut flesh, shredded.
- 3 tbsps mint, chopped.
- 1 and half cups coconut water
- 2 tbsps stevia
- Half avocado pitted and peeled.

Directions:

- In a Keep blending err, combine the coconut with the banana and the rest of the ingredients.
- Pulse well, divide into cups, and serve cold.

SALADS

Fresh Cucumber Yogurt Salad

12 Servings

Preparation time: 5 minutes

Ingredients

- 2 tbsps apple cider vinegar
- 0.5 tsp garlic powder
- 0.5 tsp ground black pepper
- 1 tsp sugar
- 1 tsp salt
- 8 tbsps Greek yogurt
- 8 large cucumbers peeled seeded and sliced
- 2 tbsps dried dill

Directions

- Place the entire Ingredient leaving out the cucumber into a bowl, and whisk this until all is incorporated. Add your cucumber slices and toss until all is well mixed.
- Let the salad chill 10 minutes in the refrigerator
- Serve.

Traditional Chickpea Salad

8 Servings

Preparation time 15 minutes

Ingredients

- Sun-dried chopped tomatoes: 24 cups
- Drained chickpeas: 2 can
- Halved cherry tomatoes: 2 cups
- Arugula: 4 cups
- Cubed pita bread: 2
- Pitted black olives: 24 cups
- 2 sliced shallot
- Cumin seeds: 24 teaspoon
- Coriander seeds: 24 teaspoon
- Chili powder: 28 teaspoon
- Chopped mint: 2 teaspoon
- Crumbled goat cheese: 8 oz.
- Pepper and salt to taste

Directions

- In a salad bowl, mix the tomatoes, chickpeas, pita bread, arugula, olives, shallot, spices, and mint.

- Stir in pepper and salt as desired to the cheese and stir.
- You can now serve the fresh Salad.

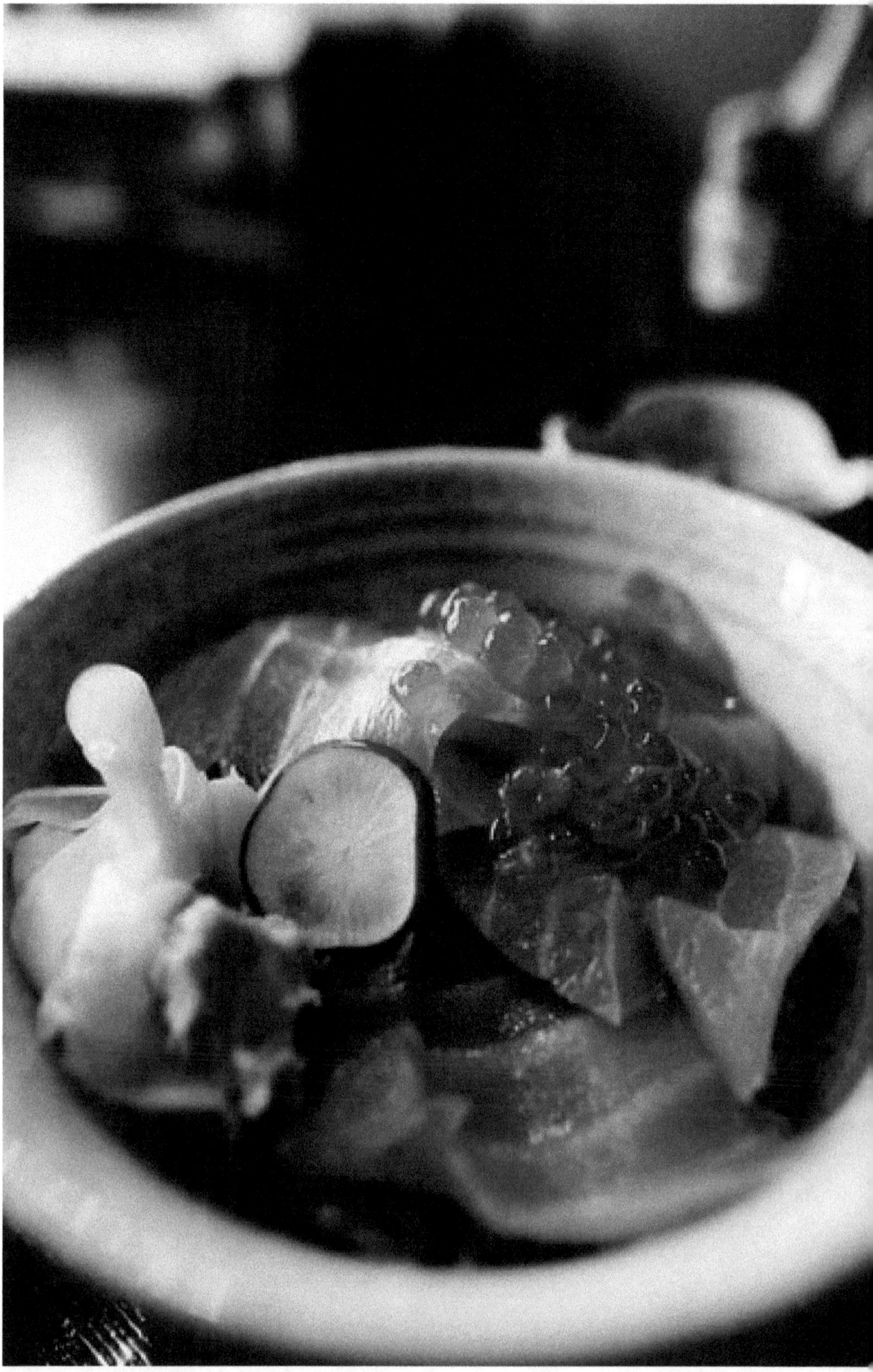

Yogurt with lettuce salad

8 Servings

Cooking Time: 20 minutes

Ingredients

- Greek yogurt: 24 cups
- Dijon mustard: 2 teaspoons
- Chili powder: 2 pinch
- Extra virgin olive oil: 4 tablespoons
- Lemon juice: 2 tablespoons
- Chopped dill: 4 tablespoons
- 8 chopped mint leaves
- Pepper and salt to taste
- Shredded Romaine lettuce: 2 heads
- Sliced cucumbers: 4
- 4 minced garlic cloves

Directions

- Mix the lettuce with the cucumbers in a salad bowl.
- Now add the yogurt, chili, mustard, lemon juice, dill, mint, garlic, and oil in a mortar with pepper and salt as desired. Then, mix well into paste; this is the dressing for the salad .
- Top the Salad with the dressing then serve fresh.

Minty Chickpea salad

12 Servings

Preparation time: 20 minutes

Ingredients

- Arugula: 4 cups
- Drained chickpeas: 2 can
- 2 sliced shallot
- Chopped Parsley: 24 cups
- Halved cherry tomatoes: 24 pounds
- Sliced green olives: 28 cups
- 2 juiced lemon
- Extra virgin olive oil: 4 tablespoons
- Chopped walnut: 24 cups
- Pepper and salt to taste
- 2 diced cucumber
- Sliced black olives:28 cups
- Chopped mint: 4 tablespoons
- Cooked and drained short pasta: 8 oz.

Directions

- Take a salad bowl and mix the chickpeas with other Ingredients

- Top with oil and lemon juice, sprinkle pepper and salt, then mix well.

- Refrigerate the Salad (can last in a sealed container for about 2 days) or serve fresh.

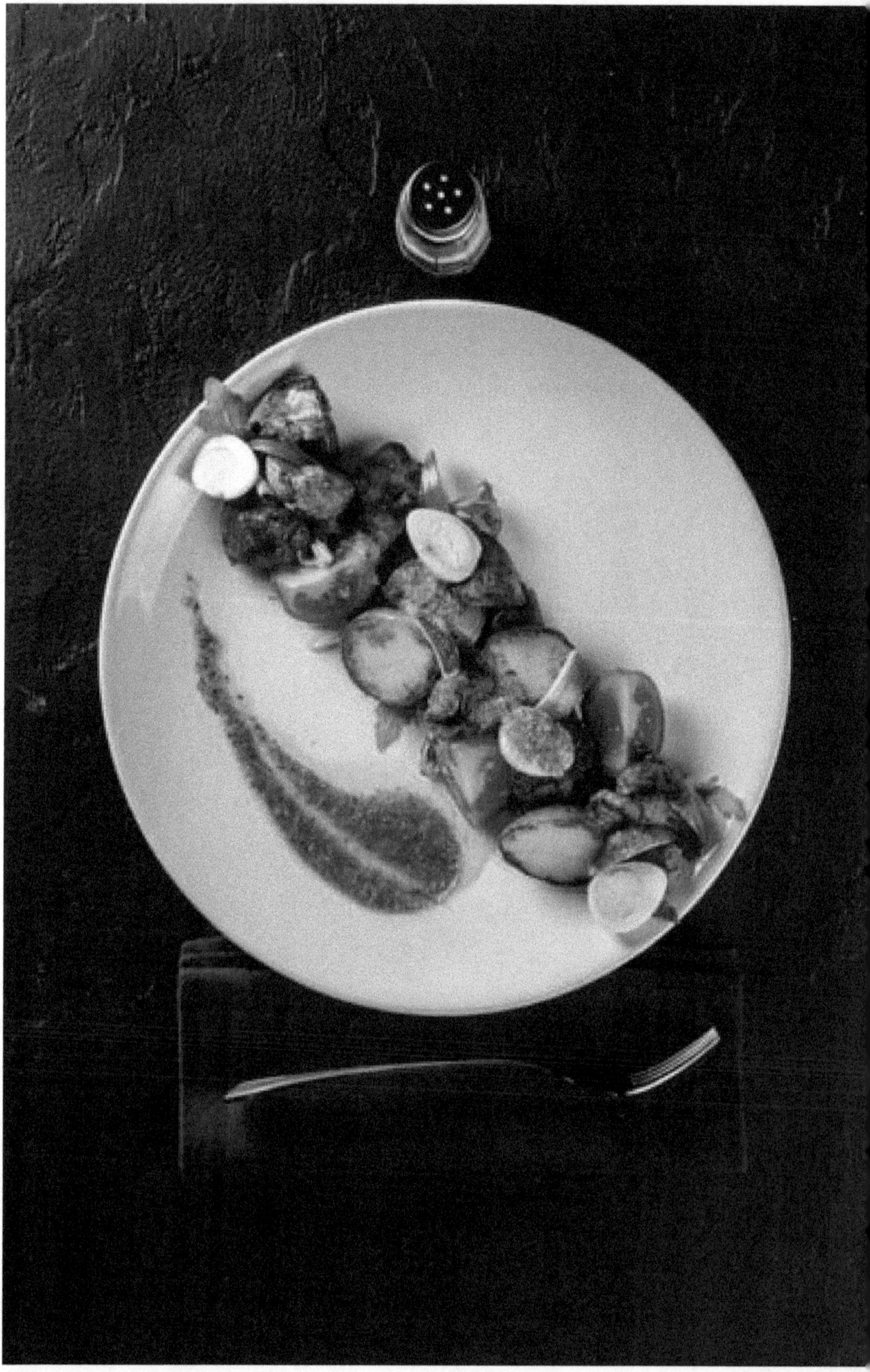

Mix Greenie salad

4 Servings

Preparation time: 15 minutes

Ingredients

- Sherry vinegar: 4 tablespoons
- Pitted Kalamata olives: 24 cups
- Almond slices: 4 tablespoons
- Parmesan shavings: 4 oz.
- Sliced Parma ham: 4 oz.
- Pepper and salt as desired
- Extra virgin olive oil: 4 tablespoons
- Mixed greens: 24 oz.
- Pitted black olives: 24 cups
- Pitted green olives: 28 cups

Directions

- Take the almonds, olives and stir there, and mixed greens together in a salad bowl
- Drizzle the oil and vinegar, then sprinkle pepper and salt as you want.
- Top with the Parma ham and parmesan shavings before serving.
- Serve and enjoy.

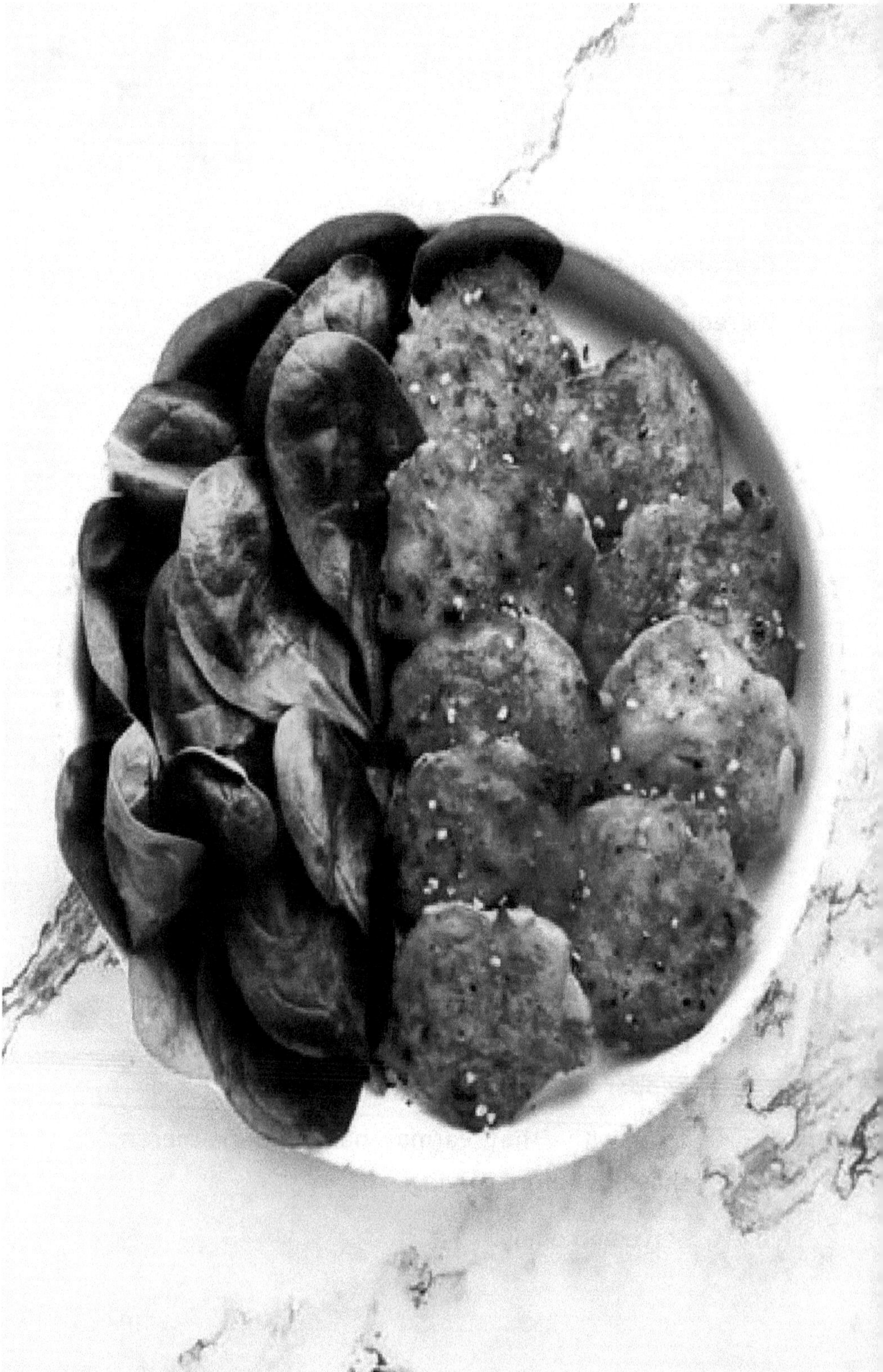

A Detox Salad

8 Servings

Preparation time: 15 minutes

Ingredients

- 2 tbsps chia seeds
- 4 tbsps almonds, chopped
- 4 tbsps lemon juice
- 4 tbsps pumpkin seed oil
- 8 cups mixed greens
- 2 large apple, diced
- 2 large beet, coarsely grated
- 2 large carrot, coarsely grated

Directions

- Except for mixed greens, combine all ingredients in a medium salad bowl thoroughly.
- Into 4 salad plates, divide the mixed greens.
- Evenly top mixed greens with the salad bowl mixture.
- Serve and enjoy

Fresh Carrot Salad

8 Servings

Preparation time: 15 minutes

Ingredients

- 2 tbsps chili powder
- 2 tbsps lemon juice
- 4 tbsps olive oil
- 6 tbsps lime juice
- 8 cups carrots, spiralized
- Salt to taste
- 0.5 tsp chipotle powder
- 2 bunch scallions, sliced
- 2 cups of cherry tomatoes, halved
- 2 large avocados, diced

Directions

- Mix and arrange avocado, cherry tomatoes, scallions and spiralized carrots in a salad bowl and Set aside.
- Whisk salt, chipotle powder, chili powder, olive oil, lemon juice, and lime juice thoroughly in a small bowl.

- Pour dressing over noodle salad. Toss to coat well.
- Serve and enjoy at room temperature.

Anchovy with Orange Salad

8 Servings

Preparation time: 20 minutes

Ingredients

- 4 tsps finely minced fennel fronds for garnish
- 6 tbsps extra virgin olive oil
- 8 small oranges, preferably blood oranges
- 12 anchovy fillets
- 2 small red onions, sliced into thin rounds
- 2 tbsps fresh lemon juice
- 0.25 tsp pepper or more to taste
- 32 oil cure Kalamata olives

Directions

- Peel off oranges, including the membrane that surrounds them.
- Slice oranges into thin circles and allow the plate to catch the orange juices.
- On the serving plate, arrange orange slices on a layer.
- Sprinkle oranges with onion, followed by olives and then anchovy fillets.
- Drizzle with oil, lemon juice, and orange juice.

- Sprinkle with pepper.
- And allow the salad to stand for 30 minutes at room temperature to allow the flavors to develop.
- To serve, garnish with fennel fronds and enjoy.